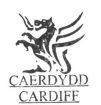
# Healthy Forever

## Connie Simmonds

The Happiest Weight Loss Book Ever!

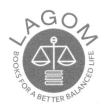

Published by Lagom
An imprint of Bonnier Publishing
The Plaza
535 Kings Road
Chelsea Harbour
London SW10 0SZ

www.bonnierpublishing.com

Hardback ISBN: 978 1 788 70036 8
eBook ISBN: 978 1 788 70037 5

A CIP catalogue of this book is available from the British Library.

Cover design by Abi Hartshorne
Content designed by Mark Golden at Crazy Monkey Creative
Food stylist: Lou Kenney
Printed and bound by Druk-Intro

1 3 5 7 9 10 8 6 4 2

Background images on pages 14, 20, 26, 32, 36, 44, 49, 55, 60, 65, 68, 75 and 85 courtesy of Shutterstock.

# Contents

# Introduction

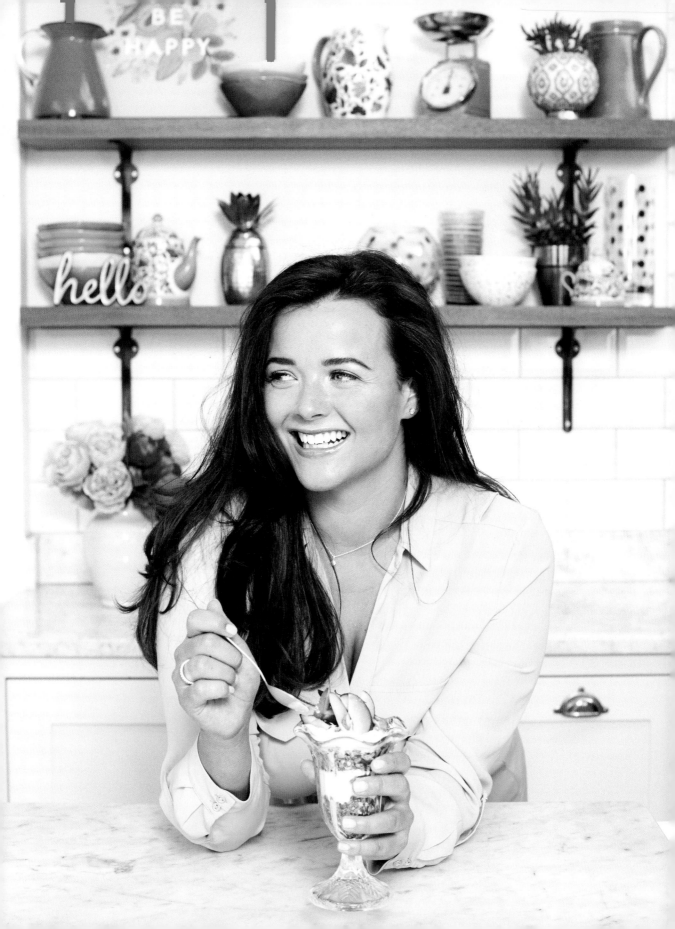

# A letter to my 16-year-old self...

Connie,

As you read this, your younger, carefree teenage years are coming to an end and you will be starting to find fault with yourself. So I'm hoping this letter will help guide you and prepare you for what lies ahead.

Between now and the age of 24 you are going to be on the most emotional, hormonal, weight-fluctuating journey of your life. But you get through it and you learn so much along the way. Just know that without the struggles, tears and constant battle to be thin, you will not go on to achieve all that you do.

Bullies will, for the first time, make you assess your physical flaws; but remember that these 'flaws' do not define you, nor do they make you any less beautiful. They become a part of your journey; they become a mark of your struggle and of your success.

From here on, you will notice the changes in your body and you will start to compare yourself to friends. Don't – you are beautiful, intelligent, strong and kind. Appreciate the diversity among you and your friends and love your body with all its curves. Take care of it, nourish it – it's the only one you will have and the more you give it, the more it will give back to you.

Believe Mum when she calls you beautiful and tells you that 'the world is your oyster' because it is true and it will rebuild your confidence. Keep your head held high, look beyond the hatred and continue to believe in yourself.

University will often get the better of you; it's actually going to be the hardest three years of your life. Food becomes your 'friend'; it is a comfort but it will also be a pain in the backside when it wants to be.

Most university students experiment with drugs, alcohol and all sorts of other things, but not you, oh no! You become an expert at experimenting with dieting, discovering all the 'tricks' of the trade, but with that come consequences. Take care of yourself; I know you are not happy in your new environment, but I wish you could see how great you look! Like so many women, you associate being slim with being happy and that's just not the answer.

Finally, you are no longer a student; you leave university with a degree in marketing, your salary is great and you've ditched the diet tablets, but now your bank statement looks more like a Time Out restaurant guide. You're struggling to find the balance between work and play; this is affecting your health and you've become quite an anxious person.

It's been two years since graduating, with two different jobs but the same bad habits: crash diets, bingeing, alcohol, eating out, denial and constant grazing. You can't find time for the gym, but really you just can't find the energy. How about trying to make it a priority? Instead of convincing yourself and everyone around you that you are happy, make a change and be honest with yourself before you cause long-term damage to your body. Masking your anxiety and insecurities with make-up and fake tan just isn't going to do it, although it does bring new success.

You become a self-taught make-up artist, featuring in showbiz magazines and gaining celebrity clients. All that practising on yourself to make you feel

> Remember who you are, what truly makes you happy and surround yourself with like-minded people.

better about the way you look has generated a whole new career path, so congratulations. Your business grows and you think you've found your calling.

With a full-time job and your own business, you seem to push your health even further to the back of your mind. Any convenient food will do: chocolate croissants, McDonalds, takeaways and junk. You've become so consumed in everything else you're doing that you've forgotten about the most important thing – your physical and mental well-being.

When does it all stop? When do you decide to become HEALTHY FOREVER in a world where it seems impossible?

Time moves on, your dress size increases and you turn what should have been a really fun family holiday into quite a miserable one. You're overweight, unhappy in your bikinis, but you're also not yourself; something is wrong. After numerous appointments with doctors, you're diagnosed with a stomach infection called Helicobacter pylori, caused by eating contaminated food or drink (you'll know exactly which dodgy takeaway was responsible as well) and the tests also flag up something that changes your mindset forever . . .

After all these years of yo-yo dieting, fat-burning tablets, tubs of ice cream, slimming clubs, over-exercising and bingeing, you never stop to consider the effect it is having on your health and the vital organs in your body. Ultimately, it is the shocking state of your health and a fatty liver diagnosis that makes you see the light. It really is a case of better late than never.

This is your true calling; this is the start of something very exciting for you. You're about to inspire thousands of women, and your passion for food, sport, female empowerment and beauty are all going to roll into one fabulously happy and healthy journey!

# Back to the Present Day

If it weren't for those results and that awful stomach infection, I wouldn't be here today, writing a book based on my journey of discovering sustainable and healthy weight loss, a journey which I'm sure many women will relate to.

**We spend so much of our time putting pressure on ourselves to lose weight for a bikini holiday or a wedding or, shockingly, a man! We often forget the most important thing . . . our health and happiness.**

I'm lucky that I valued my health enough to make a change for good; I actually had no idea how unhealthy I was until those medical results came back, but with such a strong love of life and with so much that I wanted to achieve, I got myself back up and gave my liver a run for its money – quite literally.

My biggest lesson after years of abusing my body was to start caring for it and taking the time to nourish it from the inside; after that, the outside completely took care of itself. The more I focused on what my body actually needed in order to function properly, rather than what would get me into my LBD the quickest, the more sustainable my weight loss became. This is when I decided to complete a diploma in nutrition. I've always had a real passion for food, but after understanding why and how certain foods can help and nourish us, keep us full, aid digestion and so many other amazing things, I fell in love with it all over again – and for all the right reasons!

With this book, I want to take you on a journey of realisation, offering you delicious recipe ideas and tips at every step to help make your weight-loss journey a lot more realistic, long-term and, most importantly, healthy.

It's about time we said NO to diets and YES to simple, nutritious and delicious food so that we can enjoy life at our most confident and fabulous.

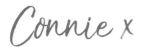

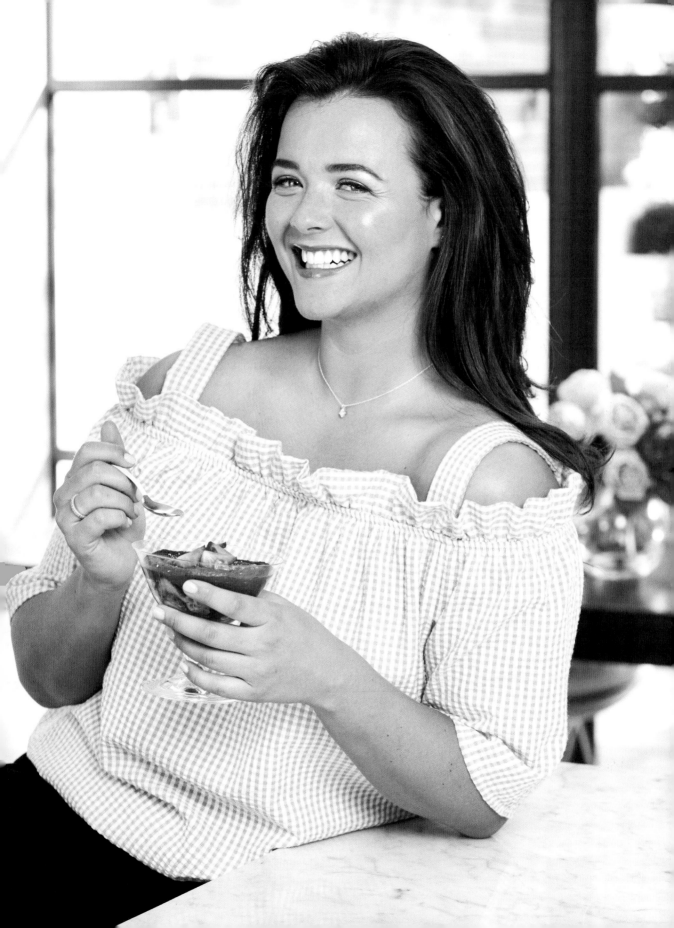

# What Made Me Change Forever

Do something today that your future self will thank you for

# My Rude Awakening

'Thank you for my results, Doctor, but just one thing: I can't understand why I've got a fatty liver.' He looked at me and, in a matter-of-fact tone, replied: 'Connie, you need to lose weight and start being healthy.' That response was the rude awakening I needed to hear in order to change things forever.

Looking back now, I'm actually quite embarrassed that I even asked the doctor that question. It's pretty clear that I was oblivious to the fact that I'd gained so much weight and to what extent it was affecting my health. Although I was focused on how I looked, that view of myself was often blurred. I may have even had mild body dysmorphia – when I was at a healthy weight I never appreciated it, and when I was overweight I didn't realise it.

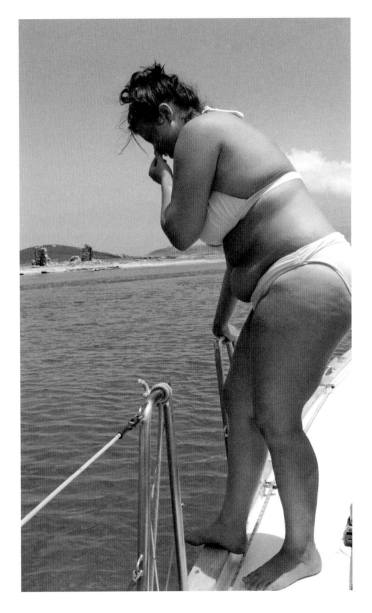

Denial was easy. My weight fluctuated so much between the ages of 16 and 24 that I lost track of what size I was and what the hell I was doing with my body. At the time I went to the doctor, I was wearing size 14 clothes but only ever wore baggy T-shirts, jumpers and leggings that stretched for miles. I was definitely avoiding the fact that I was actually a size 16, the UK's average dress size for women, but certainly not the right dress size for me.

## Anyway . . .

As I left my appointment, I got into my cute little Volkswagen UP, pretending to be okay, and just broke down crying at the wheel. My stomach felt like it was on fire because I was so furious at myself.

Two of my grandparents, both 80 at the time, had better-functioning organs than me. I looked up to them and always admired how active they were, digging away on their allotments packed full of organic vegetables and fruit. But if I admired their lifestyle so much and aspired to be like them, what was I doing about it? Nothing.

I rang my mother and said, 'Mum, good news: they've finally detected the stomach infection; bad news: I've got a fatty liver because I'm overweight.'

She was silent, then replied, 'Oh Connie that's terrible; you need to do something about it.' It wasn't one of Mum's best pieces of advice (she's usually really good), but I think she was shocked and, to be fair, she's not a doctor, so what could she say? Telling me I needed to lose weight had never worked before, so this time she opted for tough love, and who could blame her?

Mum was right. I was an adult and nobody was responsible for or in control of my health except me, so I drove home, tears rolling down my face, but, for the first time, determined to do something about it.

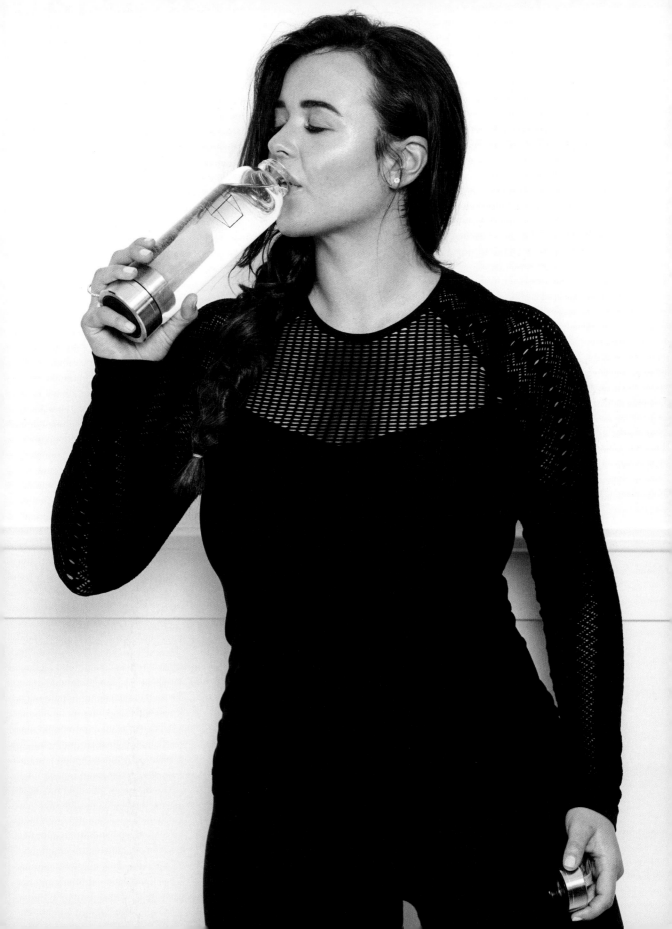

# Re-educating Myself

After going crazy on Google searching for answers, I started to notice a pattern emerging. Every credible source online (nutritionists, doctors, healthcare professionals) was recommending healthy, wholesome foods and regular exercise as a solution to my health problems.

It sounds obvious, but it took me a while to put the pieces together. Although I was determined to make proper changes, I was hoping for a quick fix, just as I always had every time I wanted to lose weight. But it didn't take me long to realise that this time things had to be different.

**If I wanted to be healthy, feel healthy and look healthy again, I had to re-educate myself and do it properly.**

Clearly, nothing I'd tried before had worked. I wasn't maintaining a healthy weight – if anything, I was expanding. But, most importantly, I realised that if I didn't change, my health issues would get a lot more serious. Being overweight can lead to heart disease, strokes and even cancer; I obviously wanted to avoid this as much as I could.

Absorbing information from actual professionals in the field was a game-changer; after all, it was an excellent doctor who opened my eyes to my obesity, so why not seek the help of healthcare professionals too? *Finally*, I saw sense.

Back at work, I took a trip to the nearest supermarket, where luckily they had a great selection of books about healthy eating. Seeing titles with words such as 'glow', 'nourish' and 'healthy' in them, I started reading and learning.

Here is how I began to re-educate myself on nutrition and healthy weight loss:
- I invested in non-biased books written by credible nutritionists/doctors who celebrated real food and a variety of it.
- I avoided books and headlines with 'diet' or 'fast' in the title. I needed to get this diet mentality out of my head.
- I disengaged with any celebrities who chose to endorse diet products promising a fast and dramatic weight loss.

By following these rules, I began my road to revival. There was one book in particular by nutritionist Amelia Freer that taught me a lot in the early stages of my journey. I learnt about the negative effects of too much sugar (before this I thought it only damaged your teeth) and I was astonished that there were such things as good fats – weren't we all told that fat-free was the key? The list goes on.

I was incredibly interested in everything I was reading and all that I was discovering, but I was also completely flabbergasted that, at my age, I had no idea about the importance of good nutrition, real food, variety and how it literally determines how we feel, think, move and look.

I believe that, as a nation, we put far too much trust in food manufacturers and supermarkets. Things may be starting to change now, but I've realised that profit is their main priority, not the customer's health. When I was growing up, the cupboards were full of processed and convenience foods: ready-made sauces, white pasta, frozen pizzas, sugar-coated cereals, and we had crisps with every packed lunch.

**Convenience foods were, and still are, highly desirable, but without a basic understanding of nutrition, it's hard to know what is and isn't healthy, especially when the packaging and branding are so persuasive.**

I decided to take matters into my own hands, to become familiar with the nutritional values on labels, to become aware of portion sizes and to shop smart. My mum has learnt so much from me and Bradley, my personal trainer brother. Although we always had fruit and vegetables growing up, she admits to grabbing anything off the supermarket shelf that looked quick and easy. And who can blame her? At the age of 24 I was doing the same and I wasn't even a busy mum with four kids who needed to be at an after-school club or football match every day of the week.

Life can be hectic, but no matter what our situation, we all need to make the most of our time. I fully understand this, but I have truly learnt that no commodity is more valuable than our health. Without good health, none of the things we become so busy with are filled with as much enjoyment, enthusiasm or happiness. Make time for your health and your health will make time for you.

Eating well is a form of self-respect

# Vanity vs Vitality

For the seven years prior to this crucial moment in my journey, I had *never* focused on my health. I had only ever focused on being skinny, dieting, quick fixes and pretty much losing weight in whatever way I possibly could. I like to think that if I had known weight loss was a natural by-product of being healthy, I might have educated myself sooner . . . or would I?

**There seems to be constant pressure on women (and men) to look a certain way, and with everything being so airbrushed and edited to perfection, it's hard to know what is and isn't real any more.**

So I think, without realising, I had succumbed to these pressures and was convinced by every beautiful celebrity-endorsed advert I saw and tried every fad diet that supermodels were supposedly doing. I remember always wanting to look like Kelly Brook, so when she lost a lot of weight through the Atkins diet, that was what I tried next. As a student, though, buying all the meat required simply wasn't affordable (and now I don't think it is good for you either). Then the TV series *TOWIE* (*The Only Way Is Essex*) started joking about 'No carbs before Marbs', and soon eating carbs became a real sin for most of us. I then saw reality TV star Jodie Marsh advertising her fat-loss pills – she had literally gone from overweight to body builder. Shockingly, after taking these I had to go to A&E with a severe allergic reaction and heart palpitations, but that still wasn't enough to stop me; the dieting continued.

I would drink a can of diet cola every morning to get my caffeine fix, and I was scanning the back of stir-fry vegetable packs to see how much carbohydrate they contained. It was getting out of control and I eventually got to my lowest point – often making myself sick after dinner because I felt too full. Now I would never claim to have had bulimia as this happened only a few times and I managed to snap out of it quite quickly, which makes me feel very fortunate. But it is safe to say that all the confusion about diets and being away from home led me to very dark times and a terrible relationship with food and my body.

My attitude was, 'If it is going to make me skinny I have to try it.' At the same time, no one in the public eye who I looked up to as a young woman was promoting real food and an active lifestyle. We were all looking for the next bullshit fad, and people were cashing in.

Now I'm not the sort of person to blame anyone for the decisions I make, because purchasing those awful pills was my choice, but I do feel that people in the limelight need to take more responsibility for what they promote and how they promote it.

If you're always on the lookout for the latest quick fix in order to shift weight fast, here's my advice:

- Change your mindset – we live in a world where everything is instant but the human body is not technology. Fast-paced innovation does not apply to us physically.
- Do not engage in any diet product endorsed by celebrities or reality TV stars without properly researching the product and its ingredients. Are you sure you want to take something you know nothing about? How do you even know that the celebrity is actually taking the product?
- Do not take diet pills, fat-loss pills or any form of tablet that claims to encourage weight loss; this is not a healthy solution and can cause long-term damage.
- Avoid skinny teas and skinny coffee as they're simply liquid laxatives; this is not a healthy way to lose weight and could adversely affect your digestive system.
- Avoid meal replacement shakes; you might be cutting out calories, but you're also starving your body of vital nutrients.

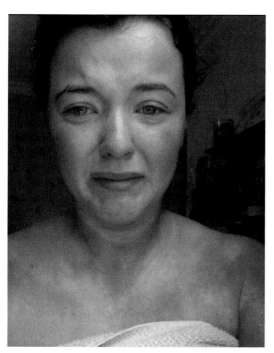

*This is a selfie I took after suffering an allergic reaction halfway through a course of those fat-loss pills recommended by a celebrity. I sent this to my family because I was away at university and just didn't know what to do.*

# Beauty Inside Out

Once I was following the right people and learning the scientific facts about nutrition, I had a little bit of an epiphany.

I was a full-time digital marketing manager for a cable manufacturing firm while running my own mobile beauty company, Cbeauty, at the weekends. Make-up, fake tan and a big blow-dry were things that had always made me feel more confident as I could hide behind the façade, so I decided to provide these services to women in the comfort of their own home. I had learnt a lot about make-up and how to spray tan at a previous job with Benefit Cosmetics, and used social media to advertise. I prided myself on being a brand that made women feel confident through grooming and the use of make-up.

However, alarm bells were ringing as I was turning the pages of my new healthy nutrition books, learning about omega 3, vitamins, minerals, amino acids and how all of these things benefit hair growth, skin health and energy, giving you that beautiful glow. All this time I had been convincing myself and my clients that gorgeous make-up was the key to confidence, yet I wasn't confident or happy myself. My back was covered with acne (which I had never suffered before) and my hair was thinning around the hairline.

Not only had I been in denial about my terrible relationship with food, but I had also been failing to acknowledge my feelings and whether or not I was actually happy.

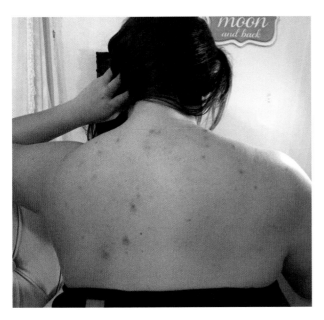

This is a picture I asked my mum to take of my back. I had come out of the shower and she noticed the large acne spots that had never been there before. I needed to see them for myself and that's why she took this picture.

I was so convincing at putting on a positive front that a lot of people continued to compliment me. I can see why – I had the big smile and fabulous make-up, and that blinded them too. People often said to me, 'You carry weight so well, it suits you.' Give me strength! I can't tell you how much that remark prevented me from losing weight. I think it is the worst thing you can say to someone who is overweight and trying to lose the excess. It's so much better to offer words of encouragement and support, especially when it's clear that they are at an unhealthy weight.

So the next part of overhauling my attitude to food was to stop promoting make-up and grooming as ways of providing clients with confidence. It just didn't sit right with me any more. I needed to rebrand and decide on a new philosophy for my business that I truly believed in.

Luckily, this was all happening at the same time that my own healthy weight-loss journey was beginning. I didn't want to shut my business down, as I love make-up and helping women feel beautiful for special occasions. But in order for me to feel happy about the message I was sharing, I felt it was right to take them on the journey with me. I wanted to share my evolution.

Beauty Inside Out was born, and I started to share all that I was learning. I began blogging and writing Instagram posts about hydration for the skin, and why great skin is the best base for flawless make-up and so forth. I was merely scratching the surface of this new way of thinking but, most importantly, I needed to put it into practice for myself.

I had adopted changes, such as reducing my refined sugar intake, which was tough, but I quickly noticed the difference that this alone made to my weight and personality. I mean, the weight loss wasn't drastic, but I could feel it starting. At first the sugar withdrawal symptoms felt like an awful head cold; it wasn't easy and I was always looking for that 4pm sugar rush with my cup of tea.

Refined sugar tastes bloody amazing, but is highly addictive, and for me the long- and short-term negative side effects began to outweigh the sugary taste itself.

As I've said before, I never knew that over-consumption of refined sugar was actually bad for your health. It wasn't until I removed it from my diet that I could really believe it.

Without getting too technical, when we eat too much refined sugar it is turned into fatty acids (fat) by the liver and spread around the body (causing weight gain). It also causes energy levels to peak and trough, and can give us headaches and cause mood swings.

## Small changes like cutting out sugar were to become vital stepping stones in how I learnt to maintain my new lifestyle.

Giving up everything at once was not going to work (I've tried that before). This time, I decided, rather than sacrificing everything I enjoyed, I would simply ensure I found healthier alternatives.

My favourite milk chocolate bars were swapped for two squares of dark chocolate, but there were occasions when I would eat a whole bar of dark chocolate because not every day was perfect and I'm not perfect. Did I still want my KitKat Chunky? Yes, of course I did! In fact, I made sure that this time I would still enjoy my favourite chocolate bar on the first day of my period – the one day of the month that nobody can stop me, not even me!

I also started making my lunches from scratch, and made time to eat breakfast in the mornings. This is when I invented my microwave egg muffins and homemade pasta sauce (see pages 94 and 128).

Mum wasn't too impressed with all the washing up (this was before I discovered one-pot wonders that keep kitchen mess to the bare minimum), but she was very impressed with my efforts to change. In fact, both my parents are amazingly supportive; they get behind whatever is going to help us become the best versions of ourselves. If you're reading this as a parent worried about your child's weight or unhealthy habits, support them in any way you can – try their food, embrace it. My whole family started enjoying my recipes with me, which acted as huge encouragement for me to carry on. They could see I had a natural flare for cooking and they were sure to give me honest feedback.

One thing I was yet to master was portion control. It is so easy to get into the mindset of thinking that because you are eating healthily, you can eat more. The other trap is thinking that because you've eaten well all week, you can binge at the weekend. I did both of these things, but I didn't give myself a hard time about it. I had to remember that I was learning and trying to break years of bad habits. Finding balance is something we are told to do, but it takes time to achieve, so don't worry if it takes a little while to get there.

One memory that does make me laugh is how I behaved around food at work (and if any of my old colleagues are reading this, they'll probably say, 'Yep, she was a feeder'). We each had two filing cabinet drawers in which everyone would have their folders neatly arranged. I, on the other hand, had all my folders on my desk so that I could make room in the filing cabinet for my new healthy snacks, porridge oats and boxes of green tea.

This is where my brother Bradley comes into play. He is a super-successful personal trainer and is now considered quite the expert, while I'm a super-proud sister. I specifically said to my mum after phoning her with my medical results, 'Do not tell Bradley or anyone about my fatty liver. I'm embarrassed but I will do something about it.' I didn't want Bradley to know because he had always encouraged me to lose weight and, more often than not, I'd declined his offers of help. Now, though, something was different. I was prepared to swallow my pride and open up to him; to stop pretending and ask for his help. Then something amazing happened!

If you want something you've never had, you've got to do something you've never done

# The Struggle and Fight Continued

Bradley was given the opportunity to write a book about life as a footballer-turned-personal trainer, with his methods and recipes. He was extremely busy with work at the time, so decided to phone me with a proposition: 'Connie, would you like to leave your job and work with me?' How ironic! I was buying all these healthy lifestyle books and now I was about to help my brother as he wrote his. I always helped him with his coursework when growing up, so it must have felt natural for him to ask me.

Without hesitation I made the decision to leave my job in marketing and work with Bradley. The timing felt perfect: I was so ready to do something new, and it would mean I could really focus on my health too.

**I was willing to halve my salary and embark on this adventure; something in my gut was telling me that it would all be worth it.**

What I forgot to mention was that, during that phone call, Bradley also said, 'You will be training with me and getting fit and healthy as part of your job role.' How bloody lucky was I? There are thousands of people who would jump for joy at the thought of training with Bradley. I, on the other hand, wanted to do it but was dreading it more than you could ever imagine. It was like a battle, a devil on one shoulder and an angel on the other. I wanted it but I knew it was going to be a long hard slog. Just because Bradley was my brother didn't make the thought of exercising my size 16 body any easier; it had been such a long time since I had consistently exercised. Anyway, I handed in my notice and that was that, there was no going back.

So I began training with Bradley. I already had my nutrition pretty much under control, so I made it very clear that if I was going to do this with him, I was not at any point going to be on a diet or start counting calories. I was simply going to eat healthy, wholesome food and a variety of it, and he agreed.

I started by doing a lot of skipping, some boxing, circuit training and HIIT (high intensity interval training). I was so heavy on my feet and was suffering terribly with shin splints. No sports bra would keep my massive boobs under control and, to be completely honest, exercise during the first couple of weeks was sheer hell.

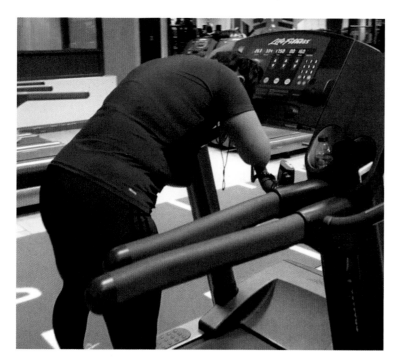

*This is the awful outfit Bradley bought me. I'm sure it would look great on the right person, but it showed what terrible shape I was in and I just felt so uncomfortable. Who would have thought it was going to be a key motivator for me?*

It was around November 2017 that it all started, so for Christmas Bradley treated me to some new workout gear in the hope that it would continue to motivate me. It was a blue-green Adidas set and my God, did I look awful in it! I felt horrible and self-conscious, but off we went to the gym. Bradley suggested filming me (he films his workouts for Instagram so that people can follow them) and I agreed. I don't know why because I looked like a whale stuffed into a condom, but I think I wanted people to see my struggle and fight. This wasn't something usually seen on social media, where most posts were made by 'perfect' people, but online realism was the one thing I lacked growing up, so others might identify with me. Then we had a light bulb moment.

## 'Let's document my journey on your Instagram feed for the next 12 weeks and show people how good you are as a personal trainer, and I can show people what it takes to lose weight for good.' Bradley responded, 'Let's do it!'

The 12-week transformation began, there was no going back. I had 200,000 of Bradley's followers watching me, but to my surprise I actually embraced the fact that so many people were tuning into my journey; it spurred me on, and the support from strangers was incredible.

Once Bradley finished editing the video and showed me, I was completely shocked and upset about how overweight I looked. 'I told you that outfit you got me was horrendous!' The video was uploaded for the world to see and Bradley became inundated with comments from people: 'Well done for helping your sister'; 'It's about time we saw someone showing how hard it is'; 'Go girl, you can do it'. I couldn't believe it, but this meant only one thing: we had to continue with regular videos and share my transformation. People wanted to see it, they were rooting for me. The pressure was on to succeed: I couldn't let them down; I couldn't let Bradley down, and, most importantly, I couldn't let myself down. But I was on fire. All the doubts, the excuses, the moaning were gone. I now wanted success more than anything.

If you've previously tried to lose weight or do gym workouts and haven't stuck to either, here's what helped me:
- Looking at old pictures of myself reminded me of unhappy and unhealthy times, and I didn't want to be that person any more.
- Buying new gym clothes that I felt confident in. I always wore comfortable high-waisted leggings, two sports bras (for maximum support) and a T-shirt.
- I told everyone what I was doing and why – some were supportive, while others didn't believe I could do it, so I turned any negative vibes into positive reinforcement.
- I took pictures along the way and compared them to the old ones so I could visualise my transformation.
- I stopped using the scales and focused on how I looked and felt.
- I pushed through the times where I felt scared or insecure; it is getting through these moments of fear that make you stronger and more determined.
- I refused to give up.

Within a couple of months I had gained 10,000 followers on Instagram. I think what made my weight-loss transformation different from others was the fact that I decided to document the actual transformation in real time; it was pretty much live footage of my workouts and daily struggles and successes. Magazines are full of transformation pictures, but nobody ever really sees the journey getting there. This was raw and personal and my new beauty inside out ethos was making more sense to my old clients and followers too.

Weeks had gone by and my fitness levels had really improved. I felt confident enough to go to boxing and spinning classes, which meant I didn't have to rely on Bradley to train me – his time was precious and I needed to know that I could do this alone. I also began training with Toni Terry, one of Bradley's clients. She was kind enough to let me join in her sessions. She loved training with others and I used her as motivation and inspiration.

One key thing I learnt through training with Toni was the importance of women supporting women. I never felt intimidated by someone fitter than me, and instead used them as motivation and inspiration. I was becoming a much happier person, I compared myself a lot less to others and was generally much more positive.

**I was training at least four times a week, eating three delicious meals a day and helping Bradley to run his business . . . for the first time in years I was happy.**

Then, in week 12, it was time to take my final transformation picture. I was all ready to post it to my followers when I began crying uncontrollably. What I had achieved was incredible and I feel proud to say that I finally loved what I saw.

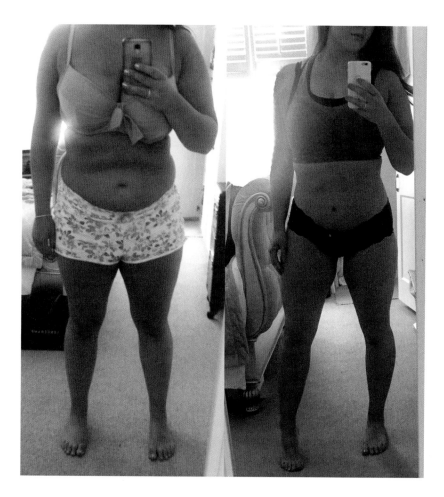

*My final transformation picture. I had dropped two dress sizes, lost a LOT of body fat, toned up my muscles without a diet pill in sight – and I was eating carbs!*

My journey so far had already inspired many people and attracted a lot of attention. Then I woke up one Sunday morning to a mountain of messages and new followers. 'Connie, you're in the *Daily Mail*,' my boyfriend Ricky said while we were lying in bed scrolling through our phones. 'Oh, yeah?' I didn't believe him, he's always winding me up and teasing me. He then showed me his phone and there I was: 'Woman drops 3 stone in just 12 weeks after a lifestyle makeover from her personal trainer brother.' I had left my job in November and by February my story was in the *Daily Mail*. I don't think I lost as much as 3 stone, but I definitely had a lifestyle makeover and I was so glad they proclaimed it in that way. That was important to me.

I later found out that the story received half a million reads and became their top story for three days running. I was on the main news page, three stories down from Jeremy Kyle and his divorce. I had to laugh. It was a serious 'pinch me' moment.

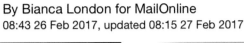

# Woman drops THREE STONE in just 12 weeks after a lifestyle makeover from her personal trainer brother who keeps premiership footballers in shape

By Bianca London for MailOnline
08:43 26 Feb 2017, updated 08:15 27 Feb 2017

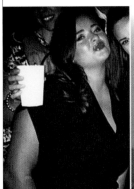
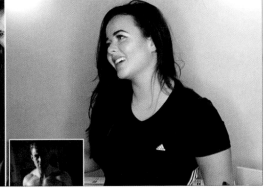

Here's the story from the Daily Mail. *People clearly wanted to know how I had done it, and thousands still assumed it was a fad or something unsustainable.*

I never read the comments from the article, but people mentioned that everyone said I'd put all the weight back on, it was unrealistic and losing weight is easy when you have a personal trainer.

None of the above is true. Since then I have lost more weight, but I've maintained my new size 12 figure. It wasn't unrealistic and the headline was just exaggerated. Of course it helps to have a personal trainer, but the commitment was all mine; I could have given up, but didn't. Nutrition plays such a huge part in losing weight too, and no personal trainer is at your constant beck and call, checking what you eat.

**All the negativity just drove me on further; I became the role model I never had when I was growing up, and that meant so much.**

*Be the person you needed when you were younger*

# The Happiest Weight Loss Book Ever

As I write this book, it has been a year since that article was published. I've continued to promote the ethos of beauty inside out and, incredibly, I've become an spokesperson for healthy weight loss. I love that I can still promote my beauty tips too.

It was a strange turn of events that led me to leave my marketing role to help Bradley write his health and lifestyle book, but nothing feels more surreal than sitting here writing my very own book. I hope this detailed insight into what made me want to get healthy forever has made you feel less alone. I hope you feel you can relate to some parts of my journey and I want you to know that if I can, you can too. I'm the girl next door – I love life, socialising, eating out and just being normal. All of this is still possible while living a healthy active lifestyle.

## *Healthy Forever* is the happiest weight loss book because I'm just like you.

I understand how demoralising it is to be continuously told how we should look, how disheartening it is to believe 'skinny' brings happiness, and how frustrating it is to try consistently yet fail on the ever-revolving wheel of fad dieting.

Though I've studied nutrition, I don't pretend to know it all when it comes to food, nor am I a personal trainer who loves going to the gym, and I'm not a celebrity motivated by money-making deals. Instead, I am someone who has truly struggled with my weight. I understand how hard it can be and now I've been given a voice, one I can use to share my journey and all that I have learnt.

I'm really passionate about helping you to achieve what I have achieved . . . a healthy, happy relationship with food.

# Where Did It All Go Wrong?

People who
love to eat
are always
the best
people

# An Irish Dancing Champion and Promising Footballer

What was it that led to my fatty liver and obesity at the age of 24? This is a question I've often had to ask myself. Do you ever find that one minute you fit into your jeans and the next minute the buttons are about to pop? I feel like it all happened just like that, so quickly and without much warning.

When my rude awakening happened and I began my lifestyle makeover, I didn't sit down and reflect on my past and what might have led to that moment; I was focused on the future. However, because I'm writing a book about my journey, I've had to dig deep. I must say it's been a truly therapeutic time and I've become so passionate about certain causes as a result, but more on that later.

I admit I've always loved my food and I'm not ashamed to say it, because loving food is definitely not a bad thing. My dad even jokes that 'more' was my first word, and I believed him! After speaking with my mum and dad, they described me growing up as an energetic, strong-minded girl with a real love of food. So what went wrong?

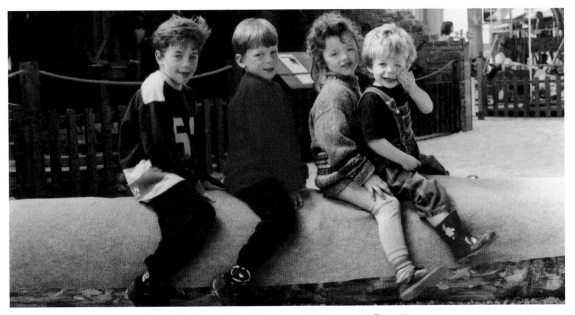

*Me with my brothers (from left to right) James, Elliott and Bradley*

Being an only girl growing up with three brothers meant I always wanted to have the same as them, do the same as them and eat the same as them. When it came to mealtimes, I remember saying things like, 'Why does Elliott have more chicken than me?' 'Why has James got the most chips?' and 'Why is Bradley's steak bigger than mine?' It wasn't even that I was being greedy, although there was certainly an element of that. I simply felt that if something was good enough for them, it was good enough for me.

Nevertheless, I loved having plastic high heels and play make-up, so mum was pleased to still have her little girl.

## From the age of five I was an Irish dancing champion, winning eight championships and absolutely loving it.

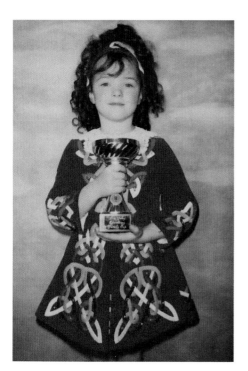

Then I got to about eleven years old and began to lose interest in the whole dancing thing, and (to Mum's dismay) turned to football. My brothers were all promising footballers at the time, so of course I had to give it a go. Turns out I was pretty good and got scouted for a professional club during a tournament in a local park. Mum became used to the idea, and, to be honest, both parents were just happy that we were all taking part in sporting activities. I think because of this I was never a chubby child. I was strong, ate well and I was positively active.

In a nutshell, then, I was a sporty child who loved her food and always had to match up to her brothers. Not much changed even when I got to high school; I continued with football, I still loved food, but I did decide to go to a different school from my brothers as I didn't want them to know my business (quite a clever tactic if you ask me). Anyway, primary school was a breeze: Mum dropped me off, picked me up, made my packed lunch, had a snack ready for me before teatime – life was bliss. Then high school slapped me in the face like a tonne of bricks.

# Periods, Pasta Pots and My PE Nightmare

On my first day at secondary school my top button was done up, my shirt was tucked in and my skirt met my knees. My curly hair was perfectly straightened with a now-vintage Babyliss straightening iron, and there wasn't a scrap of make-up on my face. But most of all, I was confident – I had existing friends around me and I was ready to take on high school. Then, weirdly, two older girls strutted over, untucked my shirt, rolled up my skirt and loosened my tie. 'That's better. You'll get bullied looking like a geek. What's your name anyway? You're so pretty, we'll look after you.' I felt special in that moment, like the chosen one, because they were clearly older. Little did I know that these girls were soon to become my high school bullies. They saw me as a threat, I think, because I walked into such a large school feeling good about myself. I was more physically developed than other Year 7 girls as I had started my periods at the age of ten, so I could probably have passed for the same age as the bullies. Unlike me, most of the other kids in my year looked too small for their uniform, so perhaps that's why these older girls saw potential in me.

My teenage years, like everyone else's, were hard enough, but at least we didn't have all the social media that exists today. There were no Kardashians or photoshopped images of unattainable perfection. We had Dream Matte Mousse Foundation and magazines.

**I can't even begin to imagine how much pressure young girls are feeling now, growing up in a world where there is always something to perceive as better than them at the swipe of a button.**

I grow increasingly concerned about this because I feel like everyone is starting to look the same and young girls are growing up way before their time. When I was a young teenager I didn't know what cellulite or stretch marks were. I was focused on sport, socialising and doing well in class so I could get a good job. Imagine what it must be like with all the pressure that exists today, on top of getting bullied? I'm not sure that even I would have had the confidence to survive that.

Back then I was a typical teenager, giving myself 45 minutes to get ready in the morning, experimenting with make-up and sacrificing breakfast for perfectly ironed hair. My blazer sleeves were rolled up and the top button was undone. By lunchtime I was starving because I'd missed breakfast, so I would eat a large pot of Pasta King (something like a Pot Noodle) and a couple of cheese slices, or a chicken burger with chips and loads of ketchup. I was always too embarrassed to get the properly cooked meals; I don't know why, but they were perceived as uncool. Looking back, I realise they would have been a lot more nutritious.

After I got my overcooked pasta and plastic cheese, I would head to the vending machines. I even figured out which machine coughed up two bags of Maltesers at a time (a fault that, much to my delight, was never fixed). Of course, everyone else was eating the same thing, so it never occurred to me to eat differently. I assumed that having a couple of vegetables at dinnertime was enough to keep healthy.

## In reality, Mum had lost all control of what I was eating; most mums probably do when their kids go to high school.

We want to be independent, and having lunch money to spend makes you feel so grown up. Because of this I wish schools would make nutrition a subject choice or somehow work it into the curriculum. I think there is so much we learn at school that could easily be dropped in favour of valuable nutrition lessons. Think about it: we eat every single day of our lives, yet nobody teaches us the importance of what we eat and why we should eat it (unless your parents are well informed, which in my time was rare). My food tech lessons consisted of baking a Victoria sponge, and I probably ate the whole damn thing!

So we've established that my schoolgirl diet wasn't great – I didn't eat a lot, but the quality and variety were poor. However, I needed no urging to get stuck into every sport possible. I was in the football team, captain of the netball team, a top-scoring discus and javelin thrower, and just loved volleyball, rounders and doing PE in general. I had a great relationship with my PE teachers and always wanted to win. Then one day an event took place that I don't think will ever leave me. It was shocking, unprofessional and completely demoralising.

By the time you get to GCSE level, PE classes are mixed (i.e. boys and girls) and I remember being on the athletics track practising for the 100 metre sprints to get into the relay team for sports day. We had a male PE teacher on this particular day, who, after guzzling down his bacon sarnie, loudly commented, 'Connie, you really need to sort out a sports bra; you can't be sprinting around like that.' I wanted the ground to swallow me up. I couldn't believe he'd say that in front of the whole class.

People sniggered and I just laughed it off, but I was mortified that he should draw attention to my boobs. I don't think I even knew what a sports bra was. At that time nobody wore them as a fashion statement, and my friends didn't need the same support as me. I went home and asked my mum to buy me a sports bra. I didn't tell her about what had happened because I was still so embarrassed. The sad thing is that when I did get into the relay team, because I was a pretty fast runner, the incident left a bad taste and took away any sense of achievement.

## I think from that moment on, I compared myself to other girls; I noticed I was curvier, which sadly made me think 'fatter'.

But I was a toned, healthy size 10. From this point onwards any negative body-related remarks played on my mind and chipped away at my confidence.

## TOP TIPS FOR STAYING CONFIDENT

1. Do *not* compare yourself to other women; we all have different DNA and completely individual biological genetics. You will never be the same as the next person, and generally that's a good thing, so learn to make the most of what you've been blessed with.

2. Feed your body with good nourishing food and stay active; it makes you feel good physically and mentally.

3. If you feel down or insecure, speak to someone, don't keep it to yourself. You're not alone in having insecurities, and remember that good friends and family will lift you up.

# Stretch Marks and Cellulite

The tips on page 41 are definitely something I would have benefited from hearing when I was a schoolgirl. Instead I kept quiet about how I was feeling and did my best to carry on as normal. Guys were still interested in me and my mum always called me beautiful, so I managed to keep an underlying level of confidence. This irritated those two school bullies though, the ones who said they'd look after me.

It was the summer holidays and if the sun was out, a group of us would get on the bus and make our way to a nearby outdoor swimming pool. Nobody cared about what bikini you had on, or if your swim shorts were designer; we were all friends having fun. Then one of the girls got a phone call, and I remember her looking at me in shock. It was the two bullies, who had heard we were at the swimming pool with the guys in their year and they started asking my friend questions about my body. 'Does Connie have cellulite?' 'Has she got any stretch marks?' 'Is she fat?' I heard it all and spent the rest of the day with a towel wrapped around me.

**I didn't know what cellulite or stretch marks were, so I casually asked my mum later that evening, which led me to scan my body for flaws in the bathroom mirror.**

It was after this episode that I started to bunk off swimming lessons, which got me temporarily kicked off the football team as a punishment. The teachers thought I was misbehaving, and for some reason I preferred them thinking badly of me than knowing the truth.

The bullying didn't just make me body conscious, it also stopped me from trusting and being open with other girls. I built up a huge barrier and I think it prevented me from making female friends easily. Those bullies affected every aspect of my school life, even my academic progress, and continued to give me a hard time right up until the day they left, which was two years before me, thank God. It meant I had two years where I was free from them and properly enjoyed school again. But the scars stayed with me.

## TOP TIPS FOR ANYONE BEING BULLIED

1.  Try to understand that bullies are often extremely unhappy or troubled, and that, putting down others makes them feel better. They get a kick out of feeling superior and feared.

2.  Speak out. I didn't tell my mum because I didn't want to worry her, but our parents are there to help.

3.  Whenever you have the chance to remove yourself from a bad situation or the wrong people, take that opportunity.

4.  Always remember that you are not alone; many people care about you, and the problem will be overcome. Stay strong.

I know now that my bullying by these girls during high school was relatively mild. Also, I wasn't isolated. Being good at sport helped me to make friends, and I could go back to a happy home at the end of every day. There I could put it all behind me and start afresh in the morning,.

**Nowadays, because of easy access to mobile phones, computers and social media, children and teenagers – and maybe even grown women – often can't escape the bullies they have to face at school, university or at work.**

It really does break my heart, so if you're reading this, you're not alone. I think you are amazing, wonderful and more than enough!

If you don't see yoursef as a winner, then you cannot perform as a winner

# From Heartbreak to Dieting

Sport isn't for everyone, and I know many people dread PE lessons. For me, however, double PE on a Wednesday morning made it my favourite day of the week. Nothing got my adrenalin pumping more than playing against rival schools in netball and football matches after hours. I was a natural-born sportswoman.

When I had to decide what A-levels I was going to study, I ticked the PE box without hesitation, but then suddenly felt a hand on my shoulder: 'Connie,' said Miss Jones, my favourite PE teacher, 'PE A-level is 90 per cent theory. You won't be doing much practical, I'm afraid.' I was heartbroken and Miss Jones knew it. She had supported me throughout my GCSE in the subject, and knew the theory side wasn't interesting to me at all. I didn't care about muscles and joints; I just wanted to win points and score goals. PE was my escape from those bullies, it was my best subject, it's where I flourished, and it was taken away from me just like that.

Now, if I gave up my gym membership, I would find an alternative way to exercise, such as HIIT classes, running, swimming or whatever. Back then, though, I didn't think, 'Oh, how am I going to exercise now?' or 'I'd better sort out my diet now that I'm not training.' I wasn't exercising or doing sport to lose weight; I was doing it because I loved it. I didn't realise how much its absence would contribute to my weight gain.

Netball finished once I reached the sixth form, as did football and all other forms of physical activity, so that we could focus on our studies. In my opinion, schools are wrong to implement this strategy. Far better to have sixth-form teams and after-school sport, something to help us unwind and get moving.

**Exercise is not only a great way to burn calories, strengthen muscles and aid mobility, but it's essential for our mood and general well-being.**

As teenagers becoming young women, we needed that release. Our bodies and hormones were all changing; we couldn't continue to eat as we had before. I had friends who felt exactly as I did about this, so we opted to take up drama just to feel like we were getting some sort of non-sedentary activity. It was never the same, and I was a terrible actress.

# MY THOUGHTS ON PHYSICAL EDUCATION IN SCHOOLS

- PE should be encouraged for every pupil, but some schools allow them to opt out if they don't fancy it. I bet they don't allow them to opt out of maths or English if they're not in the mood . . .

- After-school sport for sixth-formers should be taken more seriously by head teachers because it has obvious benefits to health and well-being.

- PE should be highlighted as something that is necessary for all human beings, not just as a school subject. It could also be linked with classes about nutrition (see my thoughts about those on page 40). The two subjects would make a great combination.

- I also think the competitive aspect of sport needs to be reinstated in schools, especially at primary level. Sport gave me my drive and determination, but had I been told everyone was a winner, what would I have had to strive for?

## So I was rid of the bullies, but then something else came along to torment me.

I didn't discover dieting as a result of a teenage heartbreak (although I did have a couple of those too). It was down to that change in the school timetable. Not long after stopping sport and taking charge of my own food choices the weight gain began. I'd say it was around the age of 17 that the yo-yo dieting began and everything started to spiral out of control.

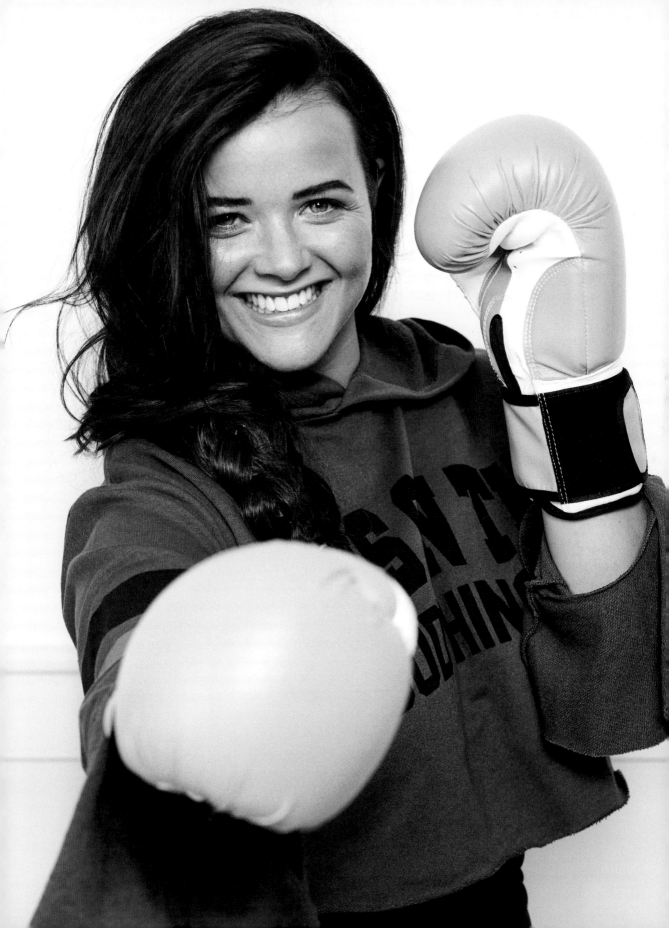

# Deli Queen

One of my first weekend jobs was working at Waitrose. I was nicknamed the Deli Queen and I loved my job because I was surrounded by the most delicious food – olives, ham, cheese, hot chickens, grilled peppers – all simply mouth-watering. I also loved interacting with the customers, slicing the meats, learning about all the cheeses. I was in my element. So much so, that when nobody was looking, I would secretly slice an extra bit of ham (usually Parma, because I have expensive tastes), and quickly shove it in my gob. When giving cheese samples to customers, I would taste with them and proclaim it was a great sales tactic. This now cracks me up. No wonder my work trousers stopped buttoning up. I probably consumed a whole joint of ham and wheel of cheese by the end of each shift.

**Something I want to highlight is that as I was no longer exercising, there was no escaping my poor diet. I firmly believe that you can't outrun a bad diet, so I'm definitely not saying that if I continued to exercise, my old eating habits would have been okay.**

For many people, obesity begins in their teenage years. I think my weight gain was just a slow and gradual one at first. I never drank fizzy or energy drinks, and we rarely had fast food or snacks at home, so my diet wasn't perfect, but it wasn't as bad as it could have been.

Then I was faced with this amazing deli counter and I was earning my own money. I started going to restaurants and drinking alcohol, and we sixth-formers were let out of school at lunchtime to shop at bakeries, supermarkets, cafés and kebab shops. When my options expanded, so did I.

### Ages 0–11
- Mum controls the food shop, what we eat and how often (she was on a tight budget with four kids, so we never overate or snacked much, fruit and vegetables were always available, and we never had deep-fried foods or fizzy drinks).

### Ages 12–15

- Mum cooks dinner for me, so breakfast and lunch are my choices, but I'm limited to sugary cereals, toast and the school canteen, plus money is tight.

### Ages 16–18

- Mum still cooks my dinners, but I have full control over my lunches, and now I'm earning money, I often go out at weekends eating and getting a taste for alcohol.

Ultimately, I would have to agree that, despite my mum's best efforts in the early days, my nutritional health definitely declined as I got older. This is because portion sizes, calories, weight gain and nutrition were never talked about at home or at school. I was completely clueless, and the only suggestions of food being healthy came from old wives' tales: 'Carrots make you see in the dark'; 'The crust makes your hair curly'; 'Fish makes you clever'; 'An apple a day keeps the doctor away'.

**I had gone from a size 10 to a size 12 quite quickly, and even began creeping into the size 14 category, depending on the style of clothing.**

I don't remember being that happy during the sixth form. It's ironic that the first time I recall being deeply unhappy in myself and with how I looked was when I began dieting.

Age fast, age slow, it's up to you

# The Diet Connoisseur

If you have no idea about nutrition, and neither do your parents or teachers, where else do you look for information? The celebrities you want to look like and the packaging on the supermarket shelves? That seems to be where I looked for it.

## FAT-FREE

The first diet I ever tried was a fat-free diet; everything I bought had to be fat-free, low fat or low calorie. What I didn't know is that not all fat is bad for us (in the right quantities) and that it naturally adds flavour and bulk to a product. Take yoghurt, for example: I now opt for full-fat bio yoghurt because it tastes better and it's the real thing. When manufacturers remove fat from products, they often replace it with sugar, artificial flavourings and sweeteners because they want it to taste just as good without the fat. However, some sweeteners can be pretty damaging to our health, and too much sugar leads to weight gain anyway, so fat-free doesn't necessarily mean better.

While following this diet, I was constantly craving sweet stuff because the sugar/ sweetener is addictive, and I was never fully satisfied because in my mind I knew I wasn't getting the real thing. This led to binges and episodes of wildly over-indulging in full-fat foods. Deprivation and restriction just weren't suitable for someone like me; in fact, they aren't suitable for anyone looking for a healthy relationship with food.

## SLIMMING CLUBS

This brings me on to slimming clubs. I've tried them and they didn't work for me: the thought of being weighed every week gave me anxiety, and counting everything I ate was unrealistic and time-consuming. I look back on it and realise that the slimming club ready meals and snacks are focused more on calories rather than nutrients and you're weirdly counting points all day. This often led me to do things like scoff loads of low-calorie chocolate bars because they allowed me to keep within my points but that isn't healthy. It also highlights how much trying to be too in control and strict with your diet can lead to you actually being completely out of control. It created a false reality when it came to how I was actually eating.

Calories are essentially the amount of energy found in food and drink, but they don't in themselves give any indication of nutritional value, such as vitamins, minerals, good fats, bad fats, proteins, fibre, etc. Calories are just calories. They are a 'simple' way of measuring food intake and ensuring that you do not eat more calories than your body needs to keep it going efficiently. However, if not done with an eye to nutritional value as well, counting calories can actually be quite damaging to your health. For example, an avocado is high in monounsaturated fat and calories, but is still very good for us, and a great alternative to saturated fats such as butter. I eat a quarter to half an avocado several days a week because of the goodness it provides, but previously I would have avoided them because they're heavy in 'points' and calories.

I felt so restricted doing the calorie-counting stuff that I ended up feeling disempowered and rebellious. As soon as I gave up on the weigh-ins (because I had lost hardly anything and felt embarrassed), I gave up all together and just put the weight back on.

**Nonetheless, slimming clubs offer a great sense of community and help a lot of people to succeed. For me, though, it isn't a long-term solution as it still sits under the diet umbrella. Weekly weigh-ins and counting points aren't real life.**

## NO CARBS

The 'no-carb diet' is similarly unrealistic. Carbohydrates are an essential part of anyone's diet. If you choose to eat the more nutritious ones (wholegrains, beans, brown rice) far more often than the white versions, you're obtaining essential fibre and B vitamins (which provide energy and prevent muscle weakness). Too many of us, myself included, became afraid of carbs, which isn't a surprise because eating mounds of white bread, pasta and jacket potatoes isn't great for anyone's health, and it's kind of all we knew. I remember thinking a giant jacket potato with tuna and mayonnaise was a well-balanced meal, just as I did a mountain of white pasta with jarred tomato sauce. As soon as I read a headline that said 'Carbs make you fat', or heard reality stars were following this no-carb method, I stopped eating them and I did lose weight.

Removing carbs from your diet *will* make you lose weight because you're reducing your calorie intake. However, by removing them, you will also reduce your energy levels, feel hungry as you'll lack fibre (which keeps you full), and be depriving yourself of a key food group, which isn't good for your mind or body. I found that it also meant I was eating too much of the other food groups, particularly dairy and protein. In fact, I became obsessed with processed meats, which aren't a healthy substitute for anything.

Something I learnt during my nutrition course was that carbs don't just provide great pre-workout energy, but they are just as essential post-workout. They help the body to restore the energy it's lost so that we can effectively carry on with our day, while the vitamins and minerals they provide aid muscle repair. It's not just proteins pumping our muscles.

Throughout my 12-week transformation, when I lost most of my excess weight, I enjoyed carbs with 90 per cent of my meals. In fact, it was during this time that I created my Loaded Sweet Potato Skins (see page 124). It was an amazing feeling to enjoy carbs again and not feel guilty about it.

## OVER-EXERCISING

When I got to university (at Bristol) I was so bored: I had no idea what to do in my spare time, and watching TV held no appeal. I tried out for the netball team (it was the A team, as I had played at county level), but I hadn't played in two years, so it soon became clear that I'd completely lost my knack. I was unfit, didn't have the right kit and felt like I had passed my sell-by date. Added to that, I got bad vibes from the other girls, who were all very serious and professional, and most of them had played for their country. There was me in baggy tracksuit bottoms and Converse. I don't think I've ever moved so fast out of a gymnasium door – quite sad really, since I used to be the last one to leave.

After going for a walk around town, I noticed a female-only gym had opened up and it was dead cheap. I liked the idea of female only, as I didn't fancy men staring at me while I was exercising. (To be honest, I was still worried about my boobs going up and down.)

## Anyway, in my spare time I went to the gym, started to lose weight and actually enjoyed it.

I then decided I would start running to the gym, do a session and walk back home uphill. If you've ever been to Bristol, you'll know how steep those roads can be. I was doing this on top of eating no carbohydrates whatsoever; this was when I was even scanning vegetables for carbs.

I drove my body into exhaustion. One day I came over all dizzy when I popped into town to take back a dress, so I headed to the supermarket across the road for a snack. I could probably have done with a sugar hit, a Snickers bar or something else sweet, but instead I picked up  a packet of . . . *cooked prawns*! What on earth was I thinking?

All I remember after that was waking up to a lovely lady in a Sainsbury's uniform telling me I had fainted and been out for about 30 minutes.

I had driven myself to collapse; my body shut down. My mum and dad were on their way to Somerset for a lovely weekend away and had to do a diversion to Bristol. When Mum saw me she exclaimed, 'Connie, you've lost so much weight!' I remember thinking, 'Yes! Goal met!' Goal met? You're in hospital after collapsing with a packet of cooked prawns in your hand. No goals whatsoever.

Exercise does offer a buzz and real sense of achievement, so I can see why people love it. However, obsession isn't something you want to achieve when it comes to exercise. What are the signs of this? Well, perhaps you feel severely guilty for missing a gym session or class and then do a double to make up for it. Or maybe you feel compelled to go for a run after every treat. Either of these mean you could be verging on obsession. If you are not allowing time for your body to rest and repair itself, you are over-exercising and doing damage.

I've finally arrived at a point in my life where I exercise because I love it and I want to do it. I've figured out what exercise styles and methods I enjoy most, what keeps me entertained, and I've continued with those.

## TOP TIPS IF YOU'RE STRUGGLING TO EXERCISE

- Try a variety of classes at the gym or in your local community, and take a friend along with you. Motivate each other.
- Make sure you are given an induction at the gym so you feel confident with the equipment and your surroundings.
- If you can afford a few personal training sessions to help get you kick-started, go for it.
- Try out new sports – boxing, swimming, horse riding, running, skipping, trampolining. There are loads out there; the gym isn't your only option.
- Go for very long walks and make a conscious effort to walk more throughout the day. This is a great start for beginners.

So I've tried multiple dieting methods, not just those discussed here, but also diet pills, supplements, soups, teas, shakes, the lot. Nothing ever led me to true happiness or self-love. I still felt fat; I felt fat for a good five years (even when I wasn't) and battled with my body and mind daily. I'm a size 12 now and by no means perfect (I still have fat) but I'm truly happy and confident and I no longer fight with myself. Being healthy has given me the courage, confidence, motivation and strength to overcome any temptation or bad thoughts I might face.

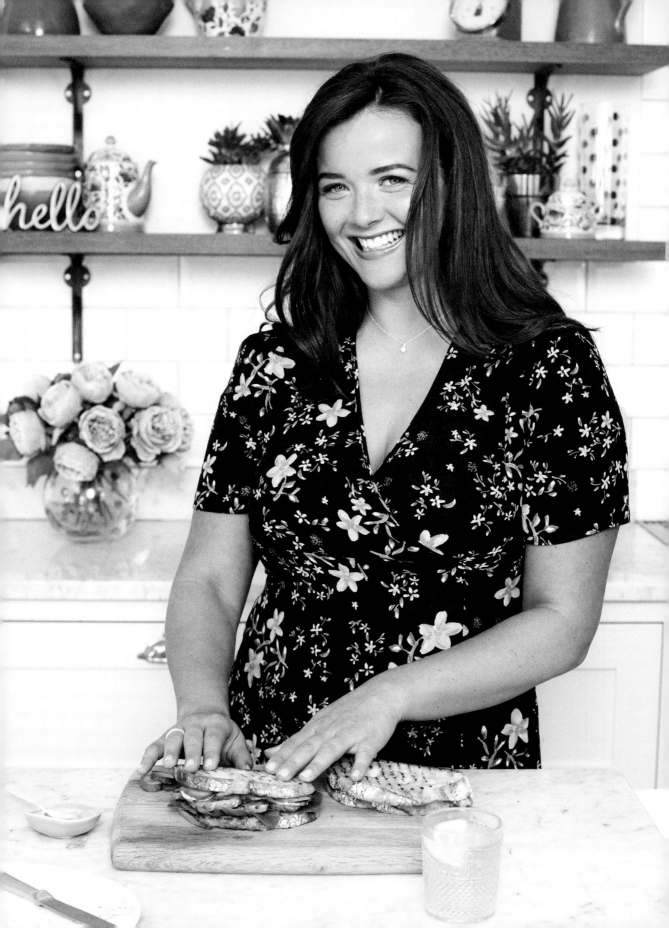

# Viewing the World Through Filters

Sadly, seeing things as they really are has become much harder in these days of social media. There is so much more influencing us, and every day we are bombarded with weight-loss adverts. We're promised the world in seven days by swallowing a slimming tablet or by drinking fat-loss shakes.

**We see hundreds of photos of men and women when scrolling through our phones on a daily basis, so comparing ourselves to others or to what we assume others look like has become nothing but ordinary in this day and age.**

We assume every image we see is real because we have faith and trust in the people we follow, but the truth is that you can never be sure.

This led me to an important decision. Just as I had taken responsibility for my own health, I also decided to take responsibility for how I was going to handle social media – as both an influencer and a user. I decided to continue showing the real and honest me, just as I did throughout my transformation, and only to follow those who inspire me, make me happy, feel good about myself and teach me things. If something isn't having a positive impact on my mental and physical well-being, I'm no longer interested.

food is love
food is life

# Grab this Book by its Cover and Go for IT

Before I tell you what my life entails now and how I continue to maintain my healthy relationship with food, remember the following:

1. You deserve to be happy and your body deserves to be healthy.

2. Any negative events that took place in the past and have led you to feel unhappy with your weight right now are over. It's time for you to move on and be 100 per cent happy again.

3. Forget anything you've learnt before about dieting and fads. Let go of it. This book is about being healthy *forever*, not for now or for a month, but *forever*.

4. This could be your opportunity to enjoy all types of food again – no counting, no restriction, no guilt, just real food and a variety of it. Grab it with both hands, take it all in and use this book as your little reminder that healthy is the way forward.

5. You will have to work at it. Taking control isn't a walk in the park, so promise me you won't be lazy, you'll take it seriously, and I promise you, you'll be so happy you did!

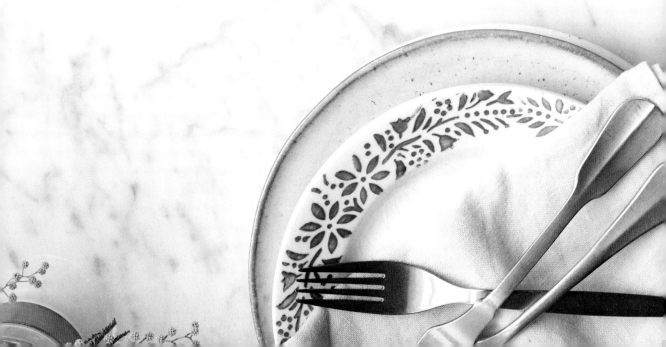

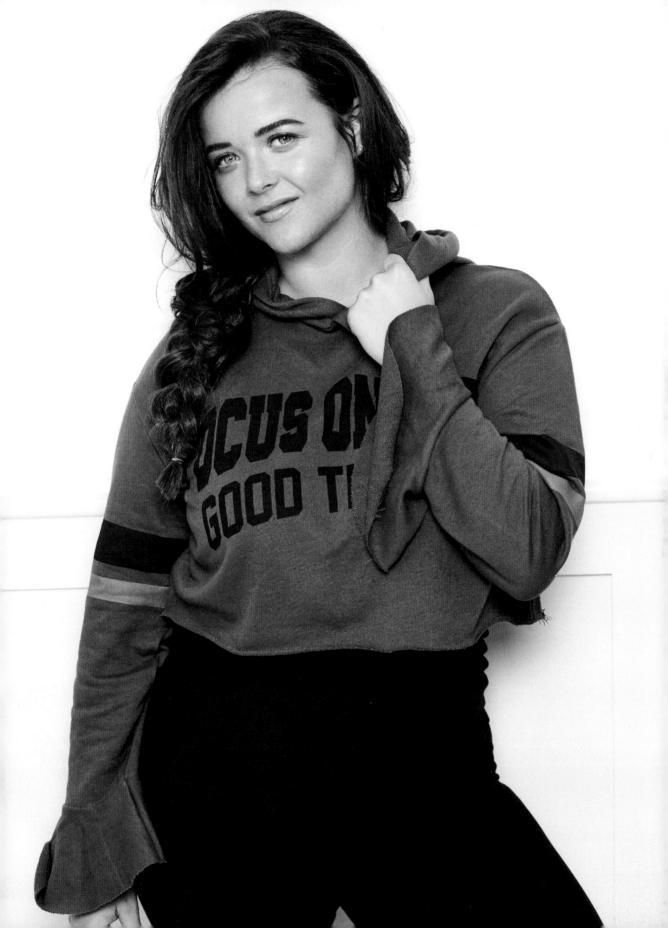

# Time To Get Started

You don't have to be great to start, but you have to start to be great

# So, Enough About Me!

This section of *Healthy Forever* is about how I can help you to become just that, healthy forever!

**What you WILL NOT be doing:**
- Losing weight as fast as you can
- Depriving yourself of certain foods
- Sacrificing your social life
- Becoming a slave to the gym

**What you WILL be doing:**
- Nourishing your body with real food
- Cooking simple meals from scratch
- Becoming mindful of what you eat and how much you eat of it
- Exercising regularly

My method is simple: eat well often, exercise regularly, be mindful of your choices and remember always to consider your health a priority.

## Just to clarify: My 12-Week Transformation

I want to be totally clear before I shed more light on the all-important next steps. I lost the bulk of my weight in the first 12 weeks of my journey. *However*, I wouldn't advise anyone to put a specific time frame on their weight-loss goals. Bradley and I simply wanted to document what was possible in a confined and specified amount of time while following a consistent fitness regime and healthy balanced diet (because fads were everywhere). The 12-week time frame has no significant importance and is not one you should necessarily apply to yourself. It just worked for me, and three months felt right for what I wanted to achieve.

We had no idea what would come of it, but at the end of the 12 weeks, my results were amazing. I had dropped two dress sizes, felt fitter than ever and my visceral fat had dropped to an amazing 4 per cent, which meant my fatty liver was healthy again. What was even better was the fact that I felt I could maintain my training schedule, and that my new eating habits became a normal part of my life. That was the best possible transformation and it has now led to this moment.

*Healthy Forever* is not a diet book . . .
Look in any dictionary and you'll find something along the lines of the following definition:

*Dieting*: *Restricting oneself to small amounts or special kinds of foods in order to lose weight.*

I strongly believe that by restricting your intake of certain foods and setting unrealistic expectations, you are less likely to stick to the changes you make and more likely to give up and revert to old habits.

Instead, I'll help you to focus on making smaller and more fulfilling changes, without restrictions, so that finding your healthy new normal is a lot more manageable, enjoyable and sustainable.

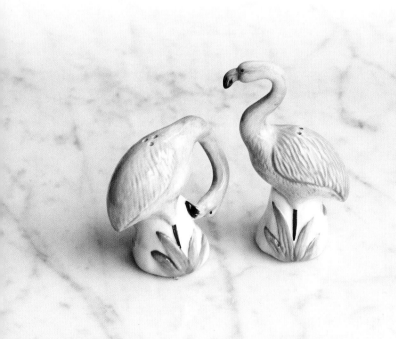

# First Vital Steps

I have faith that you've picked up this book because being healthy for the rest of your life is something you strive for. Amazing! It doesn't happen overnight and not every day will be perfect, but here are some initial steps I urge you to take in order to give yourself the best possible start.

## Open your mind . . .

By opening your mind to new ways of doing things and forgetting all that you once knew about diet and exercise, you'll find this process a lot easier.

Here's how to approach things with an open mind:
- Be honest with yourself, how you are feeling, what you are eating and the effort you are putting in.
- Don't be opposed to learning new things about nutrition or learning new skills, such as how to cook.
- Don't assume you hate something before you've even tried it; we're all adults now.
- Don't turn down help or advice from the right professionals; it could give you that extra boost of motivation and knowledge.

## Quick pep talk . . .

It is all too easy to become defensive and closed, especially when it comes to weight. It isn't really anyone else's place to tell you whether you should lose weight or not. However, the mind is a powerful thing, and the fact that you've picked up this book means it's obviously something you want to achieve. So instead of feeling embarrassed or guarded about it, feel proud, feel happy, be excited that you are going to achieve great things in the most healthy and positive way.

**If someone else has given you this book, don't be offended. Appreciate the gesture, recognise that they understand you aren't truly happy and they want you to be healthy forever because they love you.**

Remember, it wasn't until I was completely honest with myself after getting some upsetting medical results that I could then be honest with those around me, and it wasn't until that moment that I could successfully open my mind to a new outlook on healthy weight loss. That flick of the switch was a huge turning point; it gave me the strength to start again.

## Finally . . .

If your health and well-being have been pushed as far back into your mind as possible, grab them with both hands and bring them to the front, because until you start to care about your health, you'll never be 100 per cent ready for this.

I'm grateful that at the start of my journey, repairing my liver was at the forefront of my mind. It gave my weight loss a whole new purpose and meaning, one that was not ruled by time or numbers, but by my physical well-being.

This resulted in a knock-on effect, and soon afterwards everything else started to improve; Beauty Inside Out was coming to light and everything from my hair to my skin and my cellulite started to get better.

There is only so much glow that make-up can give you, and I don't think cellulite-busting creams actually work, but I'm a true believer that once you nourish and love your insides, the outside naturally looks after itself: you literally glow from the inside out. Throughout my journey, the aesthetic side of things really did blossom for me.

**If you want that flick-of-a-switch moment, consider getting a full body health scan. Maybe this will be the starting point for you too.**

- Ask your GP to refer you or advise you.
- Use private healthcare if you have it.
- Visit a nutritionist.
- Find a gym or pharmacy that has a machine for reading percentages of body fat and visceral fat, which is found around organs .
- Visit a full-body scanner (BodPod), which can read your body stats quite accurately.

# What If I Still Don't Care About My Health?

If you still don't care about your health up to this point, I'm not sure that I can actually help you. In fact, I'm not sure why you've picked up this book at all. Not caring about your health is like living a slow, painful death. It means you are refusing to face your future and the consequences of not caring for yourself. Sadly, this is something that will affect not only you, but also your family and friends.

Love yourself first because that's who you'll be spending the rest of your life with

# Spring-Clean Your Cupboards

As part of becoming healthy, you'll be eating a variety of real, nourishing food in the right portion sizes every day.

*Real Food:* *Food that is as close to its original and natural state as possible, with very few alterations, e.g. fresh or tinned tomatoes rather than additive-laden tomato sauce.*

Processed foods lack nutrients and contain additional ingredients to prolong shelf life or enhance flavour. I want you to focus on feeding your body with the most natural forms of food because that is what the body is naturally designed to consume and digest.

So now it's time to clear out your cupboards of any unhealthy processed foods, not because you can't ever eat them again, but because in these initial stages of getting healthy it is very hard to remain focused with all the temptation of old habits around you. Remove the following and donate what you can to food banks:

- Cereals high in sugar (i.e. 6g+ per 40g portion)
- Crisps
- Chocolate, sweets and biscuits
- Ready meals
- Frozen pizzas and convenience foods
- Ready-made and bottled sauces
- Fizzy drinks
- White bread or pasta

**I know I said previously that this isn't about restriction or guilt, however it is about re-educating ourselves on the importance of nourishment through real, wholesome foods.**

In my recipe section there are loads of ways to enjoy delicious, comforting sweet and savoury foods without excessive amounts of sugar, sweeteners, salt and processed sauces, so don't panic.

All of the things we've become so used to as a nation will be swapped for healthier alternatives, and you'll wonder why you didn't enjoy them sooner. There is something incredibly rewarding about cooking delicious, nutritious meals for you, your family and friends, especially when you start to see the physical results.

**A spring-clean of your cupboards and fridge-freezer is a great way to physically mark the beginning of your new lifestyle. Then you can really start to enjoy my recipes and begin writing your shopping list for the week ahead.**

### Social spring-clean . . .

I have touched on it a couple of times in previous chapters, but I just want to highlight it again because I think it is extremely important . . .

Social media is everywhere and it is an amazing platform, one that has elevated my career and allowed me to share my story. However, it isn't all roses and unicorns; it can be an extremely influential place for all the wrong reasons.

Your mental welfare is just as important as your physical, so do unfollow brands and people that make you question how you look and that tempt you into the latest diet fads or fast weight-loss solutions. They will only stump your progress and play havoc with your mind.

Social spring-cleaning is such an empowering and liberating experience, it will naturally prevent you from comparing yourself to others and will help you to avoid being caught up in the latest health and fitness trends. Instead, follow people who inspire you to be kind, happy, healthy, hard-working and anything else you feel passionate about.

**The world of social media can be a fickle place, so take it with a pinch of salt and definitely don't let it rule your life.**

What you do every day matters more than what you do every once in a while

# Smart Food Swaps

This isn't a diet book; it's about normalising new and healthier ways of eating and living while still enjoying life. I began by having a good clear-out of my kitchen cupboards; I also decided to reduce my refined sugar intake. By avoiding products with added refined sugar (check the ingredients) and swapping them for homemade bakes or fresh fruit, I was making smart changes without giving up sweet treats completely (see my chocolate and snack recipes on pages 157 and 167). I never felt I was missing out because my home bakes are amazing and I knew what damage too much sugar was doing to my body after re-educating myself on the facts about nutrition.

## The benefits of smart swaps
- Your taste buds will adapt to new flavours – which is a good thing!
- Swapping doesn't mean sacrificing flavour or enjoyment.
- You are providing your body with essential nutrients it might be lacking.

| EAT MUCH LESS OF | EAT MUCH MORE OF |
|---|---|
| Large white jacket potatoes | New potatoes or sweet potatoes |
| White pasta and rice | Wholewheat pasta, brown rice and other grains, such as quinoa |
| Creams and custards | Full-fat yoghurt with added vanilla |
| Refined sugar | Honey, dates, fresh fruit, vanilla and cinnamon |
| Ready-made sauces | Herbs and spices, tinned tomatoes, curry pastes, coconut milk, soy sauce |
| Cakes and biscuits | Quick homemade bakes |
| Processed meats and fatty cuts of meat | Chicken breast or thighs, fish, Quorn, turkey |
| Diet fizzy drinks | Fizzy water with fresh lemon and lime, or iced green tea |
| Sugary cereals and granola | Homemade granola or porridge topped with fruit and nuts |
| Crisps | Homemade crisps or a small handful of flavoured nuts |
| White bread | Seeded wholegrain bread, rye bread or fresh sourdough bread |
| Butter | Avocado or coconut oil (when baking) |

# What the Hell Is Mindfulness and How Do I Achieve It?

Even if you haven't heard of mindfulness, you have probably heard people talk about finding balance. Both of these things are pretty similar: easy to say but a lot harder to achieve. The idea is that the mind is a powerful thing and often drives us to temptation. I'm going to help you understand what it means to be mindful and why it is so important to find the strength to apply it. Here is what I understand by mindfulness:

**Knowing what is good for us physically and mentally and therefore acting upon it consistently without obsession, over-indulgence or guilt.**

For example, I know that a variety of fruit and vegetables is good for me, and I know my body needs proteins, carbohydrates, fibre, fats and water in order to function properly, so I include all these things consistently with every meal. However, I also need to feed my soul, I need to enjoy my favourite restaurants, and I need to be able to fully enjoy social situations because that is real life.

I prioritise my health every day, but once in a while, when I feel it is right, I enjoy the food and drink that we're so often told to avoid or resist – things such as ice cream, cocktails, chips, macaroni cheese, cakes and chocolate. Let's not take the fun out of food and life!

So when do I feel it is right?
- On special occasions, such as birthdays and Christmas
- On girls' nights out (once or twice a month)
- Date nights
- When I really crave something I haven't had in a while
- On the first day of my period

I never buy any of the things mentioned opposite in my weekly food shop (remember we just did a spring-clean of our cupboards); I tend to enjoy them when I'm out or socialising or, as I said, on special occasions.

When we are told we can't have something, it tends to be all we want, which is why it's such a good idea to find or make healthy alternatives. For example, if you keep some dark chocolate in the fridge, you'll find you're less likely to crave or binge on it.

I tend to remind myself that chocolate, crisps and all those other things I seem to crave aren't becoming extinct; they won't vanish off the face of the planet, so relax and put your health first.

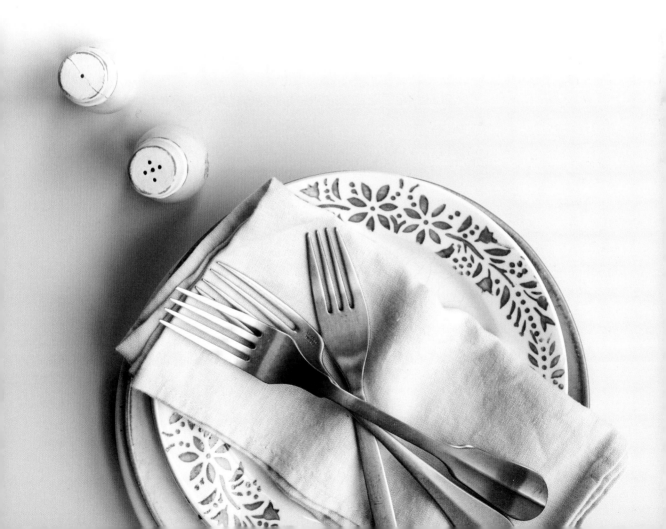

# Portion Control

Eating the right amount is a huge part of weight loss and it definitely fits under the mindfulness umbrella. Remember when I began eating better and had a filing cabinet at work full of healthy snacks? I thought it meant I could eat much more, but sadly this isn't really the case. Just because food is healthy or wholesome or made from scratch does not mean you should over-indulge in it; and if you do, don't expect to achieve amazing weight-loss results.

Initially, I do want you to focus more on making healthier choices, but you will have to accept the fact that *all* foods contain calories. As much as we want to focus on nutrient-dense foods rather than calories in order to reach our healthy weight goals, we also have to be mindful of how much of them we eat.

How I learnt to be mindful of portion sizes
- I used bowls rather than large plates when serving up my dinner – this prevented me from piling on too much food.
- I ensured every food group was included, but in the right quantities. (Although when it comes to vegetables, I'm not fussy about amounts.)
- I discovered what was officially classed as a portion size for all the food groups; for example, a portion of chicken or turkey is about a palm-sized amount.
- I stopped eating just for the sake of eating and instead focused on building a balanced plate of food at every mealtime in order to keep me fuller for longer.

Initially, getting portion sizes right will be a bit hit and miss. I struggled with this at first, but once I had overcome that hurdle, things became easier. I eventually discovered that snacking wasn't something I needed to do. Three meals a day with plenty of water was enough for me. The only time I tend to snack now is if there are large gaps in between meals or if I am bored, so I always make sure there are healthy options to hand for those moments (because boredom often gets the better of me).

All my recipes in this book indicate whether the recipe makes one, two or more servings, so you already have helpful guidance on what a portion should look like; many of them also include serving suggestions.

# Cheat Days and Meals

I advise you to erase the concept of cheating from your life. It contradicts everything you are trying to achieve when building a healthy lifestyle without fads and binges.

Cheating on your body by eating lots of refined sugar and fatty foods isn't really going to achieve anything other than headaches, energy slumps and delayed feelings of guilt.

**I used to think food made me happy, but actually it's the social and family aspect of food that I really love. It's the discovery of new flavour combinations and watching others smile as they enjoy my food that brings me happiness. Not cheat days.**

A cheat day is essentially a day to binge and that isn't right. It's not about creating a healthy relationship with food – it screams BINGE as a CONSEQUENCE of DEPRIVATION, and that is certainly not what we want.

Instead, refer back to what I said about mindfulness (see page 70). Occasionally enjoying foods that I love, but that aren't necessarily high in nutritional value, is not something I assign to a particular day (unless it's something like a birthday or Christmas tradition), and it is not something I force myself to do.

Nevertheless, there are bound to be days when one thing leads to another and you'll feel like you're falling off the wagon. So overleaf you'll find my tips on how to get back on it without feeling guilty.

# Falling Off the Wagon and How to Get Back On

1. Being honest about falling off the wagon is the first step. It's important to know and admit when you've reverted to old habits so that you can stop and restart.

2. Never fall off the wagon for longer than necessary; just jump back on!

3. Never wait for Monday to get back on the wagon (this is a very common mistake); make it your next meal or snack. Don't let whole days go by or, even worse, weeks.

4. Don't feel guilty about it; life is too short. A bad food day isn't going to ruin your life. Get over it and remember all that you've learnt and why you started.

**Alcohol and eating out . . .**

In 2017, more and more of us were choosing to exercise with friends. I love this trend and I really hope it sticks. I think finding new ways to socialise with friends that doesn't involve alcohol is such a positive thing.

I've made many new friends as a result of my new lifestyle, and it's great to have different friends for different activities. For example, my training friends and I often have a healthy post-workout breakfast together, while with other friends I enjoy an occasional slap-up meal and cocktail.

**Alcohol is never really going to have a positive impact on any person's weight-loss journey. Not only is alcohol itself often high in sugar (and therefore calories), but the inevitable hangover the next day often means craving salty, greasy foods.**

I also suffer with anxiety after consuming too much alcohol, and this was a major factor in reducing my alcohol intake. I now drink alcohol about once a month and I really enjoy myself. I haven't had anxiety from alcohol since making these changes.

Nowadays, my favourite night with friends is to cook them a three-course meal, complete with candles and music to set the scene. And, of course, a few cocktails to start the evening! That's why I had to include some healthier cocktails in this book (see pages 191–5).

**What I love about this approach to losing weight and keeping it off is that without a stressful time limit or strict rules to follow, I never felt under pressure when I hit a bump.**

I knew that if I was doing what was good for me most of the time, then a bump in the road wasn't going to ruin my progress. Having this relationship with food again and not feeling like I was breaking the rules of a strict diet brought me a sense of calm and relief.

Eat healthily, sleep well, breathe deeply, enjoy life

# Exercise

Fitting in exercise is often the biggest concern people have, especially if family, multiple jobs and other commitments reduce the amount of free time you have.

**If you already feel like you're up to your eyeballs with work and home life, here are five steps to getting your head around fitting in exercise:**

1.  Plan and organise each week at a time: food, exercise, socialising, chores.

2.  Prioritise exercise on certain days (see it as something that can't be sacrificed).

3.  Exercise does not have to be time-consuming to be effective. Thirty minutes of HIIT, bodyweight or circuit training is better than nothing.

4.  You can't outrun a bad diet, so keep your nutrition in check.

5.  Incorporate exercise into your family life by going for long walks or play time in the park. Or why not exercise at home once the kids are in bed?

A lot of people will say that losing weight and living a healthy lifestyle is down to 80 per cent nutrition and 20 per cent exercise. I understand this, but for me those percentages make exercise seem unimportant.

If it weren't for exercise, I wouldn't feel as strong, sexy, confident and fit as I do now. Exercise gives a different sense of accomplishment and satisfaction than I get from eating well. I have found my passion for sport again because of how empowered I feel at the end of a session. When people say you never regret a workout, they're not wrong.

In reality, exercise not only aids your weight loss, it also helps you to tone up while you lose the weight. I think it prevented me from getting saggy skin on my arms and stomach – areas that all too easily suffer this problem after weight loss alone. Also, after strengthening my core muscles, the back pain I was suffering with disappeared.

So if you want to feel strong, fit, sexy, confident and empowered, I highly recommend you to find out what exercise you love and go for it.

Here's how . . .
- Try every type of exercise class possible until you find the ones you enjoy.
- Join a gym that offers unlimited free classes with your membership.
- Invest in several sessions with a personal trainer to learn the ropes.
- See what is happening in your community, e.g. running clubs and zumba classes.

My favourite exercise and classes are:
- Boxing gyms or 1-2-1 boxing
- Circuit training with others
- Spin classes with pumping music
- Running, if I need to unwind and think

What do I do if I'm not motivated?
I definitely don't love the gym and exercising as much as, say, working with a personal trainer. There are days when I just don't have the motivation to do it. However, if I have planned a class and it's in my diary, I never cancel. If I plan to meet someone for a gym session, I never cancel. The only time I am likely to back out of exercise is if it is not properly scheduled – in other words, if it isn't planned in advance and is inconvenient. So my advice would be:

- Join a gym where you can go with people who encourage you to work hard.
- When you book classes, commit to them. Don't cancel except for a real emergency.
- Exercise at a gym or community centre that is near home or work so it's convenient for you to get there.
- Plan your workouts for the week so you can get the most out of them. (You can find so much inspiration online; check out @bradleysimmonds on Instagram.)

To be quite honest, sometimes you just have to cut the bullshit and get on with it. A class might only be 45 minutes, which is no time at all, but it will be 45 minutes that you won't regret; 45 minutes of hard work with the most rewarding results.

Gym starter kit
1. A good pair of high-waisted, squat-proof leggings
2. A supportive sports bra (regardless of your size, you must protect your assets!)
3. Proper gym trainers (suitable for running)
4. A padlock for the locker (otherwise you'll be dragging your bag around with you)
5. A bottle of water (stay hydrated)

You can find lots of advice on my favourite things by following my Instagram page @conniesimmonds – I'm always happy to help!

# Food

Before we head to my delicious recipes in the next section, I want to highlight some tips around shopping for food and drink.

The most important thing for me to say is that there are no rest days when it comes to good nutrition. For the remainder of your life you want to be enjoying foods that are nourishing for the body, mind and soul! And don't forget – that does include those occasional takeaways, glasses of wine and slices of cake (but remember, be mindful).

Smarter swaps will eventually be things you naturally pick off the shelf because small changes like these are easy to adopt. Eating a variety of real food is easy to do as long as you re-educate yourself and get a little organised.

Here's how . . .

1.  Do your food shopping online: it allows you to visualise your trolley more clearly and you're less likely to be distracted into buying processed foods.

2.  Eat a variety of colours when it comes to fruit and vegetables.

3.  Enjoy a variety of food from all the important food groups (see opposite).

4.  Follow the qualified nutritionists and doctors on social media who share their nutritional know-how and tips.

5.  Keep this book close so that you have healthy recipes readily available – even ones that don't require cooking!

## The five important food groups . . .

I find that knowing *why* you are being told to eat or drink something makes you more likely to consciously do so again. Once I learnt about the different food groups and why they are *all* essential for the human body, I became a lot less scared about eating them, and every plate of food then had significant nutritional value.

| FOOD GROUP | WHY IT IS IMPORTANT | SOURCES |
|---|---|---|
| PROTEIN | Proteins are essential building blocks of the human body. Your body needs them in order to repair and rebuild. It also needs protein to make enzymes, hormones and other body chemicals. Your hair and nails are made mostly of protein. | Animal sources, such as meat, poultry, fish, eggs, milk, cheese and yoghurt. It's also found in soy products (tofu), Quorn, nuts, seeds, beans, and grains such as quinoa. Vegetarians and vegans must be a lot more conscious of their protein intake: quality vegan/non-vegan protein powders are a great addition to diets lacking in protein. |
| CARBOHYDRATES | The body's main source of energy comes from carbohydrates. The best types are those containing lots of fibre, as they take longer to digest, keeping you fuller for longer and providing you with more nutrients than the more processed kinds. | Wholegrains, quinoa, potatoes, oats, brown rice, beans, pulses, rye bread and other wholegrain breads. White bread, pasta and rice are stripped of these fibres and nutrients, making them a less healthy choice. This doesn't apply to white potatoes, though. |
| FATS | There are different types of fat: unsaturated (good) fat provides the body with essential fatty acids (omega 3) and helps it to absorb vitamins such as A, D, E and K. Too much fat of any kind will hinder weight loss, but some fat in your diet is essential. Unsaturated fats can also help to reduce cholesterol levels and reduce the risk of heart disease. | Oily fish (e.g. mackerel, salmon trout), nuts, avocados, olive oil. |

| FOOD GROUP | WHY IT IS IMPORTANT | SOURCES |
|---|---|---|
| VITAMINS & MINERALS | Together, vitamins and minerals form the most essential nutrients for the human body. With deficiencies in any of them, the body simply does not function properly. Vitamins and minerals help to boost the immune system, heal wounds and repair cellular damage. They simply feed the body with goodness. | It is very important to get the right amount and right variety of vitamins and minerals into the body. You can do this by eating a range of foods, particularly fruits and vegetables, which carry them in abundance. I believe that vegetables in particular should be eaten with every meal. The best way to ensure you are getting an adequate intake of vitamins and minerals is to eat fruit and veg in a variety of colours, not just green! |
| DAIRY | Food containing milk or milk products is high in calcium, which is essential for maintaining healthy bones. It also provides us with a good range of vitamins (particularly B12) and other minerals (including magnesium, phosphorus and zinc). | Milk, yoghurt and cheese. However, if you are dairy-intolerant, you can find calcium and other essential vitamins and minerals in lots of fruit and vegetables, and in eggs, tofu, hazelnuts and chickpeas. Do your research and seek professional advice. You might need additional supplements, but this must be advised by a doctor or registered nutritionist. |

## My before and after shopping list . . .

Here are some examples of what I used to buy in my weekly shop in comparison to what I buy now. Can you spot the difference?

| BEFORE | AFTER |
|---|---|
| White penne pasta | Broccoli |
| White rice | Mixed peppers |
| Stir-fry vegetables | Pak choi |
| Stir-fry sauces | Asparagus |
| Chicken breasts | Avocados |
| Prawns | Edamame beans |
| Pork chops | Garden peas |
| Big bag of cheesy Doritos | Red onions |
| Large bar of Galaxy chocolate | Sweet potatoes |
| 6-pack of Diet Coke | New potatoes |
| Crunchy Nut Cornflakes | Spring onions |
| Full-fat milk | Carrots |
| Potatoes | Aubergine |
| Onions | Tomatoes |
| Gravy granules | Mixed fresh or frozen berries |
| Ketchup | Bananas |
| Mayonnaise | Mixed salad leaves |
| Sausages | Chicken breasts or thighs |
| Bacon | Salmon fillets |
| Thick white sliced bread | Fillet steak |
| Butter | Chicken sausages |
| Chocolate Müller Corner yoghurts | Trimmed bacon |
| Beef mince | Quorn mince |
| Ready-made pasta sauce | Full-fat bio yoghurt |
| Garlic | Almond or coconut milk |
| Mushrooms | Vanilla grinder or extract |
| Peppers | Fresh garlic and ginger |
| Chocolate digestives | Chillies |
| Cheddar cheese | Coconut oil |
| Nutella | Olive oil |
| Crunchy peanut butter | Balsamic vinegar |
| Melt-in-the-middle chocolate puddings | Honey |
| Ice cream | Parmesan cheese |
| Olive oil | Goat's cheese |
| Frozen pastries | Dark chocolate (70% cocoa solids) |
| Fresh orange juice | Selection of nuts and seeds |
| Ham and garlic sausage | High-quality nut butter |
| | Mixture of flavoured rice pouches |
| | Kidney beans or mixed beans |
| | Fresh or frozen herbs |
| | Oats |

You'll see that in my previous shopping list I still had lots of healthy, wholesome foods but not enough of them, and definitely not enough variety. I was also eating processed meats, ready-made sauces and sweets far too often. Most of the sweet stuff that I enjoy now is whipped up quickly using natural ingredients, and my food is flavoured with herbs and spices instead of artificial flavours and excessive amounts of salt and sugar.

Now here is an interesting insight to a food day in the life of me. You can see an example of what I used to eat and what I would eat now.

| THEN | NOW |
|---|---|
| **BREAKFAST**<br><br>2 slices of seeded toast with butter and Marmite<br>1 Diet Coke or shop-bought fruit smoothie | **BREAKFAST**<br><br>2 tbsp full-fat natural yoghurt<br>2 tbsp homemade granola<br>1 handful of chopped berries<br>1 cup of ordinary tea without sugar, or green tea |
| **LUNCH**<br><br>1 large burrito packed with cheese, chicken, salsa, soured cream, salad, jalepeños<br>1 Diet Coke<br>2 chocolate-covered rice cakes<br>Maybe a packet of crisps or sweet-and-salty popcorn | **LUNCH**<br><br>1 chicken breast, sliced and seasoned with Cajun spices<br>1 wholemeal wrap<br>½ avocado smashed and spread on top<br>Mixed salad and jalapeños<br>Large glass of no-added-sugar summer fruit squash |
| **DINNER**<br><br>Big bowl of spaghetti bolognese, using white pasta and topped with a good handful of mature Cheddar cheese<br>Anything sweet I could find in the cupboards, usually some biscuits<br><br>I also drank water throughout the day. | **DINNER**<br><br>Smaller bowl of spaghetti bolognese, using a 50/50 mixture of wholewheat pasta and courgetti topped with homemade sauce based on lean beef or turkey mince, and a sprinkle of Parmesan cheese<br>2 squares of dark chilli chocolate.<br><br>I drink water throughout the day. |

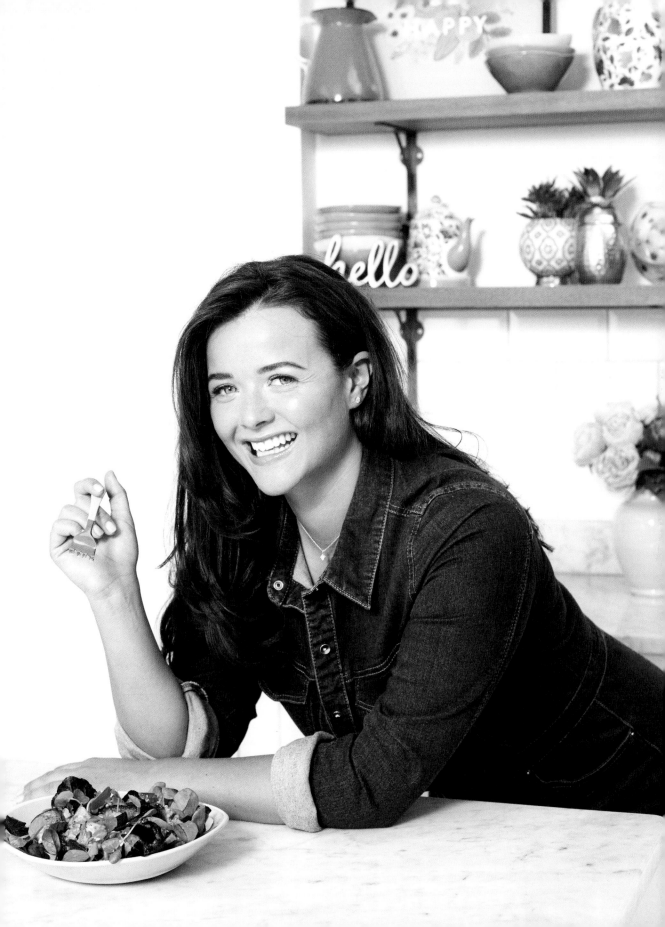

# Hurdles Along the Way

Whether you're 3 weeks, 12 weeks or 12 months into making the changes outlined in this book, there will be hurdles and setbacks along the way. On some days you will lack motivation, on others you will eat too much, and that feeling of frustration for not getting instant results might creep up on you.

However, if you follow my advice using the steps given in this section, the results will appear more quickly than you think, and they will be results that you will be able to sustain and feel completely proud of.

Just always remember why you started, and never lose sight of your long-term goals and your long-term health.

# It's time to be happy and healthy forever!

Stop looking for happiness in the same place you lost it

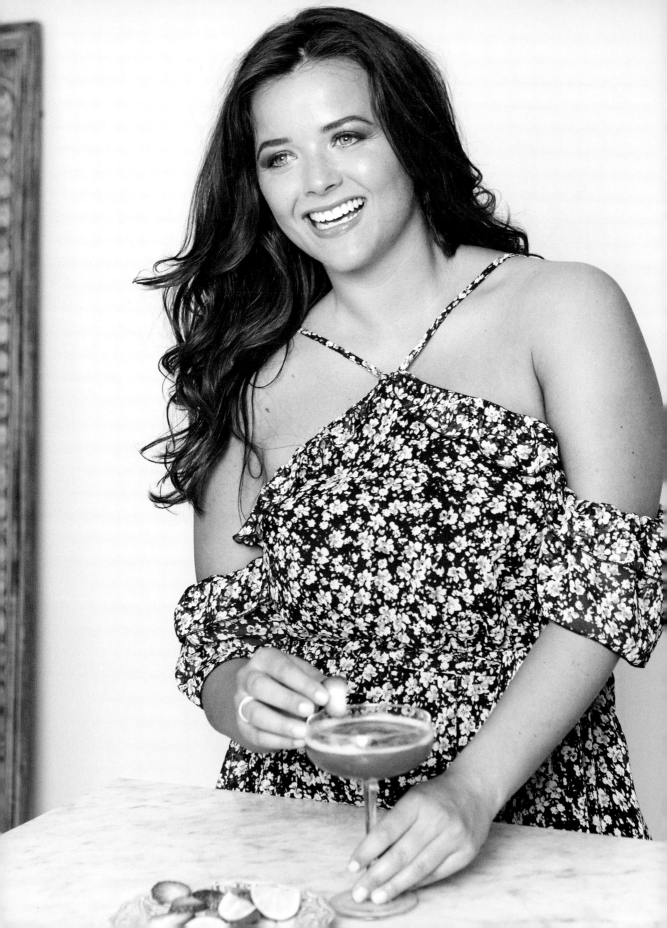

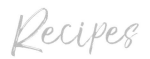
# Recipes

As you've probably guessed, I've always been a foodie; my mum said that even as a toddler I was always willing to try new food. Aged three, she caught me in the pet aisle of the supermarket tucking into a tin of cat food, so I certainly wasn't a fussy eater.

**Luckily, as I've got older, my taste in food has vastly improved, and so has my nutritional knowledge.**

Having started out completely unaware of how much damage too much of the wrong food was having on my body, I now really appreciate unprocessed food, balanced meals and colourfully varied plates. Alongside that, I'll still enjoy a little of what I fancy, and have found clever ways to turn my unhealthy favourites into much healthier versions.

**All of this has enabled me to lose weight, sustain my weight loss and feel happy, energised and a lot more confident in my own skin.**

**Finally,** no more fad diets, fear of missing out, bingeing or feeling hungry!

BEFORE YOU START ON THE RECIPES THAT FOLLOW, HERE ARE SOME KITCHEN ESSENTIALS AND INGREDIENTS YOU WILL NEED
(all other recipe ingredients can easily be found in your local supermarket)

- Spiraliser and/or good vegetable peeler
- Good blender
- Ground almonds – a great alternative to flour
- Ground flaxseed – because it is high in omega 3 and adds bulk to dishes
- Vanilla grinder or good-quality vanilla extract – one of my favourite alternatives to sugar, as it provides natural sweetness
- Chia seeds – because they are high in protein, fibre and omega 3

# Breakfast

Start your day with the right attitude and the right breakfast.
I find that my breakfast sets the tone for the rest of the day,
but I often get bored with the same old thing and need options that are
quick to prepare but still delicious and filling. These recipes will become
your morning lifesavers; you'll feel energised and ready
to take on the day with a belly full of fuel.

# Morning Berry 'Cheesecake'

This wholesome breakfast is creamy and fruity without the guilt and – even better – it's made the night before so you can wake up to a delicious breakfast that feels almost too good to be true. I tend to make mine in a portable plastic container or jar because it's such a great breakfast to eat on the go.

## All you'll need: (serves 1)

50g rolled oats

1 tbsp chia seeds

4 tbsp natural full-fat yoghurt

Large handful of frozen mixed berries

Several chopped nuts to sprinkle

## Method:

1. Starting with the oats and chia seeds, layer up your ingredients, adding them to a flat-bottomed container.

2. Then spoon in the yoghurt, spreading it evenly across the oats.

3. Sprinkle your frozen berries over the top and finish with the nuts.

4. Cover with some cling film or a lid and leave in the fridge overnight.

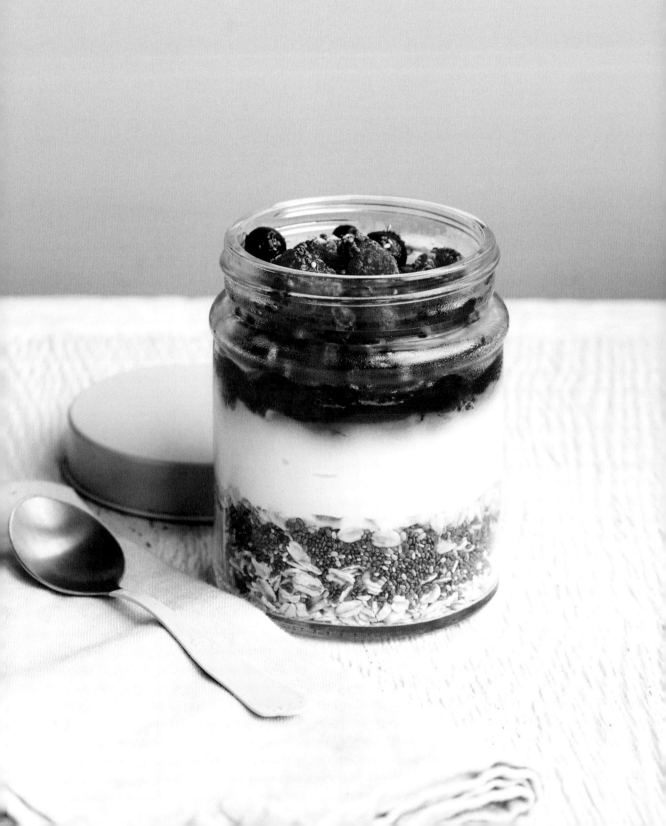

# Healthy Hash Browns Topped with Avocado & Runny Egg

A big thing for me when losing weight was to make sure that at no point did I feel I was missing out. So I discovered ways to create healthier alternatives to the things I loved, like these hash browns. Team them with some good fats and lean protein and you're on to a winner.

**All you'll need: (serves 1)**

**For the hash brown:**

1 medium white potato (150g)

Drizzle of olive oil

Salt and pepper

**For the toppings:**

½ avocado, sliced

1 free-range egg, poached

Splash of Tabasco (optional)

**Method:**

1. Preheat the oven to 200°C/gas mark 6 and line a baking tray with greaseproof paper.

2. Clean the potato, then grate using the large holes of a cheese grater (you can peel the potato if you wish, but there is no harm in including the skin).

3. Add the grated potato to a bowl with a pinch of salt and stir, then form into a pattie-like shape. I don't like mine too thick as it takes longer to cook, so aim for about 2cm .

4. Place the hash brown pattie on the lined tray, brush with some olive oil and season with salt and pepper.

5. Pop in the oven to bake for about 30 minutes (flipping over halfway through). Some ovens might take longer, but ideally you want a golden finish.

6. Top your hash brown with sliced avocado and a perfect poached egg (see page 96). Season with salt and pepper and add a splash of Tabasco, if liked.

You can prepare the hash browns in bigger batches and freeze them (uncooked) for whenever you're ready to bake them.

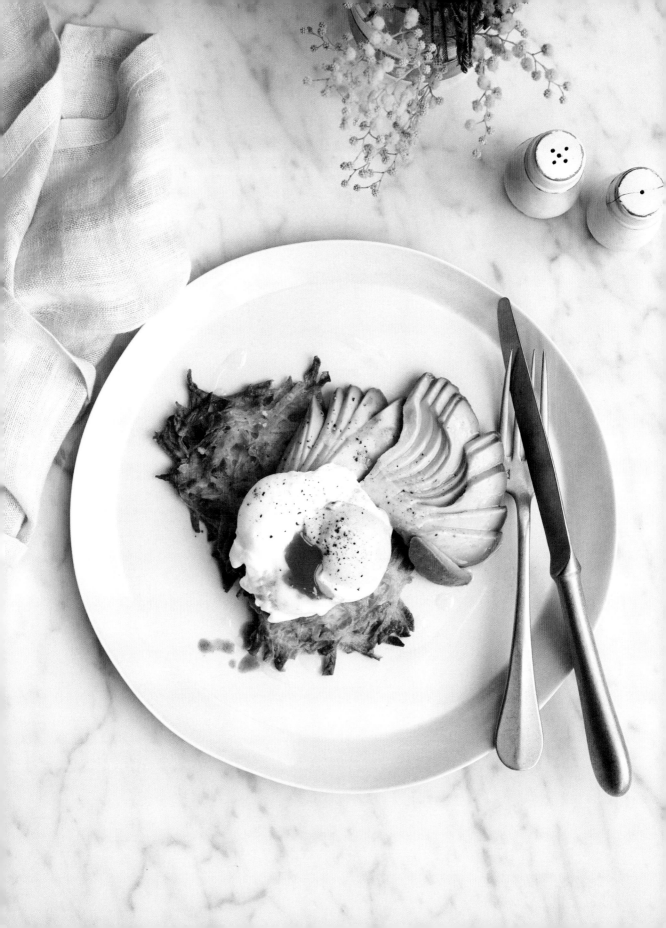

# Minute Egg Mug Muffins with Avocado, Tomato & Spring Onion

These little protein-packed gems are ideal for a quick breakfast without all the fuss. I used to make them in mugs in the office microwave because it meant I was never late and never hungry!

I'd advise at least two egg muffins per person with a slice of rye bread to ensure you're getting all your essential carbs and fibre.

**All you'll need: (makes 2)**

Oil for brushing or drizzling

2 free-range eggs

2 splashes of milk

¼ avocado, chopped

4 cherry tomatoes, halved

1 spring onion, chopped

1 tsp ground turmeric

Salt and pepper

**Method:**

1. Drizzle or brush 2 microwavable mugs with some olive oil.

2. Crack an egg into each mug, then distribute the remaining ingredients equally between the two and whisk with a fork.

3. Pop in the microwave for 30 seconds on a high setting, stir and then heat again for another 30–40 seconds until the egg is fluffy and set in the mug.

4. Feel free to sit at your desk and eat straight out of the mugs, or empty the egg muffins onto a plate and eat with a slice of toasted rye.

You can vary the fillings: I recommend any sort of veggies, such as peppers, mushrooms, courgettes or spinach, and instead of avocado you could sprinkle in some feta or goat's cheese. Jalapeños or chilli flakes work really well for flavour and spice – the options are endless.

# Home-Baked Nutty Granola & Peach Sundae

Now this is a beautiful breakfast or brunch, and you can go super-fancy with how you serve it, making it the perfect coffee morning showstopper. I like to stack it up when friends are round, otherwise I simply sprinkle it into a bowl to enjoy all on my own. I particularly love this recipe because it combines my low-sugar homemade granola with my favourite fruit: peaches.

**V**

**GF**

**All you'll need:**

**For the granola: (this makes a batch for the week, so you can enjoy it for several days)**

250g rolled oats

4 tbsp honey

2 tbsp melted coconut oil

100g mixed nuts, chopped

1 tbsp vanilla extract

2 tsp ground cinnamon

**For the rest: (serves 1)**

1 peach or nectarine, stoned and
   sliced into segments

Greek or full-fat natural yoghurt

Chopped pistachio nuts, to sprinkle

**Method:**

1. Preheat the oven to 180°C/gas mark 4 and have a baking tray ready.

2. Add all the granola ingredients to a bowl and mix with clean hands or a wooden spoon. It will be sticky, so just make sure the honey and coconut oil are coating the oats and nuts as evenly as possible.

3. Spread the mixture evenly across the tray and bake in the oven for 7 minutes until lightly toasted.

4. Remove the baking tray and turn the oven off, but put the peaches onto another tray and pop into the still-warm oven; this allows them to gently bake and caramelise nicely while the granola cools.

5. Once the granola is cool, start layering up your yummy sundae with granola, peaches and yoghurt. Finish with a sprinkling of pistachio nuts.

Both peaches and nectarines are great sources of vitamins (such as B, C, E and K) and minerals (such as potassium, calcium and magnesium), all essential for muscle, bone and heart health. However, you can add whatever fruit or nuts you like to this versatile recipe.

# Halloumi & Homemade Pesto with Roasted Tomatoes on Toast

Now I won't lie to you: I discovered this amazing flavour combination at a gorgeous healthy café and I just had to recreate it. It's great for when you have a little more time on your hands and fancy something hot, savoury and meat-free.

## All you'll need: (serves 2)

### For the nut-free pesto:

¼ avocado

4 basil leaves (I don't like my pesto too strong so feel free to add more), plus a few extra for garnish (optional)

1 small garlic clove

Juice of ½ lemon

Drizzle of olive oil, if needed

### For the rest:

2 large tomatoes, halved

4 slices of halloumi

2 free-range eggs

2 slices of sourdough bread

Salt and pepper

## Method:

1. Preheat the oven to 200°C/gas mark 6 and line a baking tray with foil.

2. Put the tomatoes (cut side up) on the lined tray, season with salt and pepper and add the halloumi slices. Pop these into the oven to roast while you prepare the eggs and pesto (10 minutes should be more than enough time).

3. Add all the pesto ingredients to a blender (or use a bowl and hand blender) and blitz until the mixture has a nice liquid consistency, adding the oil if needed; set aside.

4. Now poach your eggs: half-fill a deep frying pan with water and place over a medium heat. Once the water starts to bubble, crack your eggs into the pan as if you were frying an egg. Let the eggs poach in the water nice and gently for no more than a couple of minutes, then turn off heat. While the eggs are poaching, toast the bread.

5. Top the toast with a drizzle of pesto, then the roasted halloumi and tomatoes followed by the soft-yolk egg. Feel free to drizzle a little more pesto over the top and garnish with extra basil leaves (if liked). Enjoy!

Any leftover pesto can be added to a salad dressing, or used in a sauce with chicken.

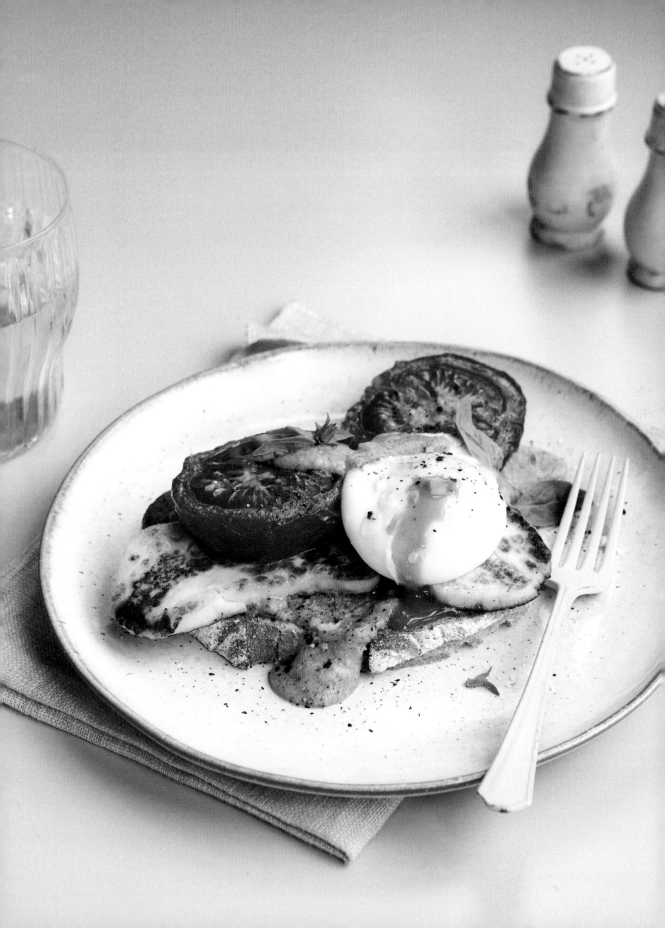

# Five-Minute Crêpes with Chopped Banana & Strawberries

I've tried so many 'healthy' pancake recipes, I thought I had been put off for life, but then I made these light, nutty crêpes so quickly and with very few ingredients that I was won over. They're really simple: just five minutes of cooking and no dodgy pancake flipping – just delicious morning crêpes.

### All you'll need: (makes 2)

3 tbsp ground almonds

2 large free-range eggs

1 tsp vanilla extract

Oil for frying

½ banana, chopped

6 strawberries, hulled and chopped

Dollop of natural yoghurt

### Method:

1. Add the ground almonds, eggs and vanilla to a bowl with a splash of water and whisk to create a smooth batter.

2. Heat a teaspoon of oil in a non-stick frying pan and then pour in half of the batter mix, ensuring it's evenly distributed in a circular shape. Gently cook for 1 minute on each side. Transfer to a plate and keep warm.

3. Repeat this with the rest of the mixture so that you have 2 golden brown almond crêpes.

4. Top with the banana, strawberries and yoghurt and enjoy.

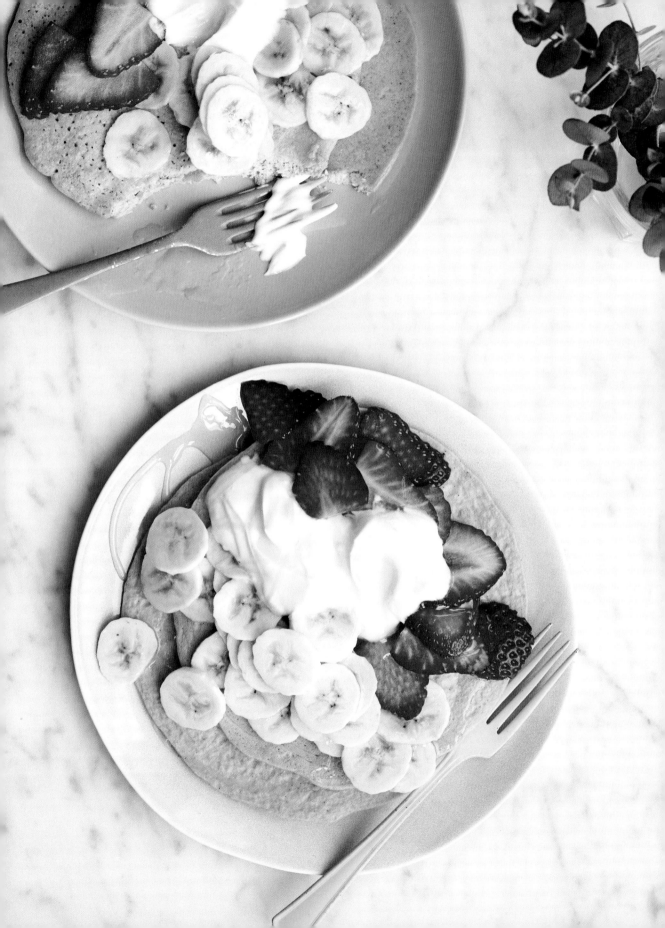

# Banana & Blueberry Grab & Go Muffins

These beauties are simply delicious with a comforting cup of your favourite tea. They're far better to grab and go than any pastry, and they're completely free of refined sugar. From baby cousins to grandparents, the whole family loves them!

**All you'll need: (makes 12–14 muffins)**

450g rolled oats

2 tbsp ground flaxseed (optional)

2 free-range eggs

2 ripe bananas, mashed

125g blueberries

1 tbsp olive oil or melted coconut oil

100ml milk (any type)

2 tsp baking powder

2 tsp ground cinnamon

1 tsp vanilla extract

½ tsp salt

**Method:**

1. Preheat the oven to 180°C/gas mark 4 and line a muffin tray with paper cases.

2. Blitz 350g of the oats in a blender to create a flour-like consistency, then tip into a mixing bowl.

3. Add all of the other ingredients and mix to make a batter. Don't squash the blueberries too much (you could keep some aside and add them whole at the end).

4. Spoon the batter equally into the muffin cases and bake for 20–25 minutes.

# Orange & Almond Overnight Bircher Muesli

I love this zesty breakfast because it is packed full of radiance-boosting ingredients, such as flaxseed, orange zest, oats and almonds. Also rich in omega 3, vitamin C and proteins, this little wonder is a breakfast fit for a goddess.

**All you'll need: (serves 2)**

70g rolled oats

2 tbsp linseed/flaxseed or chia seeds

Zest of ½ orange, plus a few orange segments (optional)

175g full-fat natural yoghurt

10 chopped almonds

**Method:**

1. Add the oats, seeds and orange zest to a bowl and mix together. Pour over 300ml boiling water and leave overnight.

2. The next day stir in three-quarters of the yoghurt and spoon into glasses or bowls.

3. Feel free to top with orange segments from the zested orange, then add another spoonful of the remaining yoghurt and sprinkle on the almonds for extra crunch and goodness.

This Bircher muesli can include any fruit of your choice. I love adding fresh cherries to mine as they work so well with the orange and almond flavours and are packed full of essential vitamins and minerals.

# My BEAUT Bacon Sandwich

I do love a bacon sandwich and figured that if I had to give up all the food I enjoyed, sustaining my new healthy lifestyle would be too difficult. So I've simply tweaked the classic bacon sandwich to become a more beautifying one.

## All you'll need: (serves 1)

2 rashers of bacon (pork or turkey), fat trimmed off

4 slices of tomato

Splash of Worcestershire sauce

2 slices of rye or sourdough bread

½ avocado, mashed or sliced

Small handful of spinach leaves

Salt and pepper

## Method:

1. Add the bacon to a non-stick frying pan (no oil necessary) and place over a medium heat, turning the rashers after 2 minutes. Once flipped, add the tomato slices with a splash of Worcestershire sauce (only on the tomatoes) and let sizzle for another minute or so.

2. In the meantime, pop the bread into the toaster and prepare the avocado – I like to season my mashed avocado with salt and pepper.

3. Spread the avocado on one of the slices of toast, top with your cooked bacon and tomatoes, and finish off with spinach leaves and the final slice of toast.

4. I squish it together to let the flavours infuse, slice it in half and get stuck in.

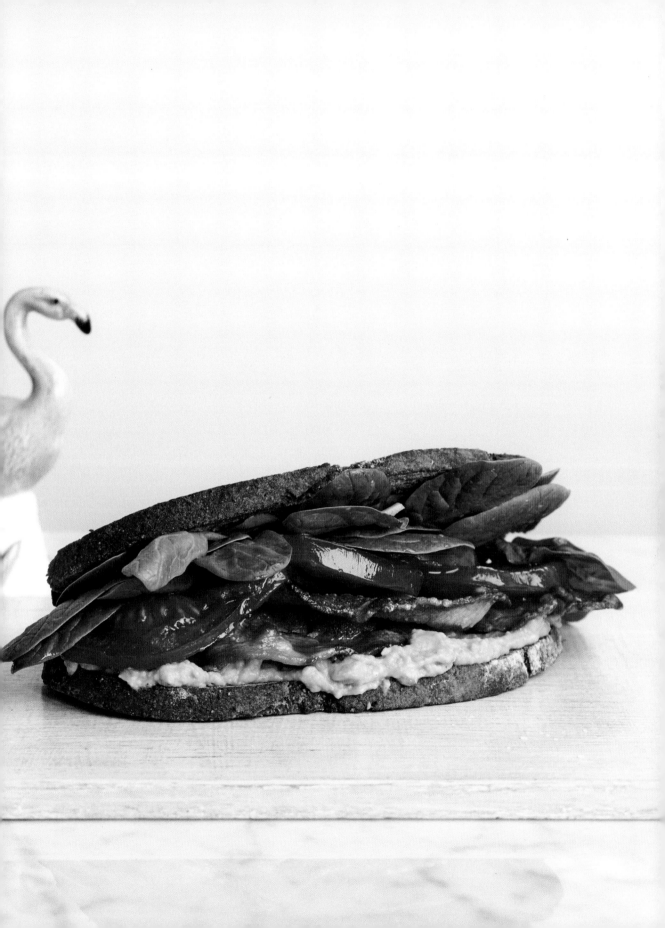

# Omega 3 Sunshine Smoothie

During my studies, I learnt about the importance of omega 3, an essential fatty acid that significantly aids the health of our heart, brain, bones, muscles... the list goes on. It also helps the body to burn any stores of excess fat, so every day I try to ensure I get my recommended daily allowance of omega 3. This delicious smoothie is one of the ways you can do it without having to think about it too much; just bung it in a blender and blitz.

**All you'll need: (makes 2 big smoothies)**

Handful of spinach leaves

1 tbsp ground or whole flaxseed

Thumb-sized piece of fresh ginger, peeled

1 tbsp oats

½ avocado

50g strawberries

1 kiwi

300ml water or coconut water

4 ice cubes

**Method:**

1.  Add the spinach, flaxseed and ginger to the blender and blitz to a pulp. Then add the rest of the ingredients and blitz until smooth.

2.  If you hate bits, you can pass the smoothie through a sieve, but there is a lot of goodness and fibre in those bits, so try not to remove them if you can help it.

# Coconut & Raspberry Porridge

Coconut is one of my favourite flavours; I find it quite indulgent and creamy, and it's also high in HDL (good cholesterol), so it makes the perfect porridge, especially when teamed with sweet and sharp antioxidant - rich raspberries.

**All you'll need: (serves 1)**

50g rolled oats

300ml coconut milk

2 tsp chia seeds

Vanilla extract

50g fresh raspberries

1 tbsp desiccated coconut (optional)

Drizzle of honey

**Method:**

1. Add the oats, milk and chia seeds to a bowl and microwave for 1 minute, then stir together. Feel free to add a splash more milk to get the consistency you like.

2. Add at least 1 teaspoon of vanilla extract and stir in; this gives the mixture a subtle sweetness and comforting flavour.

3. Top with raspberries, desiccated coconut, if liked, and a drizzle of honey.

# Lunch

Deciding what to have for lunch can often be a task in itself, especially when your days are full to the brim. I've been a 9–5 office worker, poor university student and make-up artist on the go, driving here, there and everywhere with only fast food restaurants in sight.

So I've thought up an array of gorgeous and colourful lunch recipes that can be made the night before and put together with ingredients that certainly won't break the bank.

Convenient food doesn't have to mean junk food; it just requires a little thought and organisation, and believe me, the options that follow all taste better than any supermarket sandwich!

# Red Thai Salmon Burger with Cucumber & Carrot Ribbons

I'm a sucker for Thai food; I think it's my favourite cuisine after good old comforting British food. These fragrant and moreish salmon burgers are my clever way of marrying the two cuisines together while getting that all-important oily fish into my diet.

## All you'll need: (serves 4)

### For the burgers:

4 skinless salmon fillets, cut into chunks

2 tbsp red Thai curry paste

1 spring onion, chopped

Thumb-sized piece of fresh ginger, peeled and grated

1 tsp soy sauce

Small bunch of coriander, finely chopped, plus extra leaves to garnish (optional)

1 tsp olive oil

### For the rest:

2 pouches of ready-cooked wholegrain rice

1 cucumber, peeled into ribbons

1 carrot, peeled into ribbons

1 lemon, cut into wedges

## Method:

1. Add all the salmon burger ingredients, except the oil, to a blender or food processor and pulse until roughly minced – you still want a nice coarse texture.

2. Tip out the mixture and shape into 4 equal burgers.

3. Heat the oil in a frying pan over a medium heat and fry the burgers for 4–5 minutes on each side, turning them once, until golden and crisp.

4. Pop the rice pouches in the microwave to heat through while you prepare the cucumber and carrot.

5. Once everything is cooked, pop each burger on top of a bed of rice, garnish with the cucumber, carrot and coriander leaves (if using), adding 1 or 2 lemon wedges to squeeze over the top.

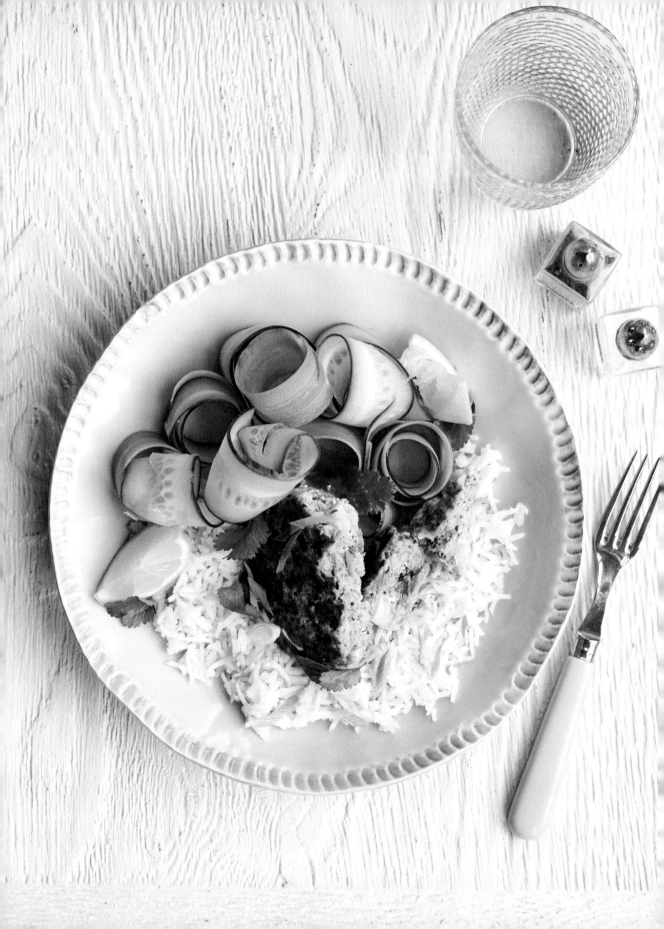

# Quick Pitta Pizzas

Now, a pitta bread's sole purpose shouldn't be simply for dipping. Not only does it act as the perfect pouch for fillings, it also makes the ideal base for my super-quick and easy 'pizzas'. I prefer these little boats of cheesy goodness warm and straight from the grill, but who doesn't also love cold pizza?

(V)

**All you'll need: (serves 2)**

2 wholemeal pitta breads

2 tsp tomato purée

4 slices of tomato

½ chopped spring onion

Handful of spinach leaves

25g mature Cheddar cheese

2 basil leaves, torn

**Method:**

1. Preheat the oven to 180°C/gas mark 6 and place a baking sheet or tray in the oven to heat up.

2. Spread the pittas with the tomato purée and top with the tomato slices, spring onion and spinach.

3. Transfer to the hot baking sheet and bake for 10 minutes until the purée is bubbling and the veggies have browned. Meanwhile, preheat the grill to high.

4. Sprinkle over the cheese and pop under the grill until the cheese has melted.

5. Scatter over the basil leaves for that real Italian taste.

You can in fact add whatever veggies you want to these pizzas. I love topping mine with jalapeño chillies.

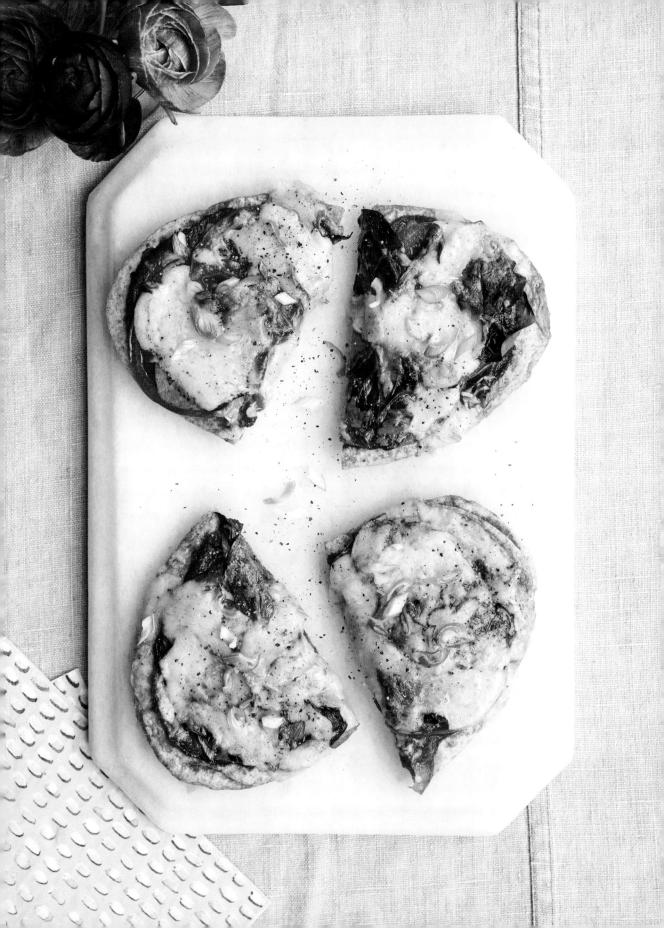

# Britain's Favourite Chicken Tikka Pockets

Asian food has fantastic flavour, so using curry paste to marinate chicken works a real treat. With chicken tikka masala being Britain's most popular dish, I had to include it in a delicious yet nutritious recipe for everyone to enjoy.

**All you'll need: (serves 1)**

1 chicken breast

1 tsp tikka masala paste (check the label to make sure it has no added sugar)

1 large wholemeal pitta

Handful of spinach leaves

4 tsp tzatziki (shop-bought is absolutely fine)

**Method:**

1. Preheat the oven to 200°C/gas mark 6.

2. Cut the chicken into strips and toss into a bowl with the tikka masala paste. Stir to coat the chicken and set aside to marinate for as long as possible before arranging on a baking tray. Bake in the oven for 20 minutes.

3. Cut the pitta in half and pop the two halves into the toaster so that they go a bit crispy (you don't want floppy pittas).

4. Gently open up the pocket in each pitta and stuff some of the spinach leaves into each one. These line the pitta and help to prevent any drips.

5. Spoon 2 teaspoons of tzatziki into each pocket and then pop in equal amounts of chicken. Lunch is served.

# Minute Steak Sandwich with Onions & Pickles

Can you believe there is a steak sandwich in my weight-loss book? This is a gorgeous weekend treat and ideal post workout. When you're in a tough gym session, just remember you're going home to enjoy this mouthwatering sandwich of champs!

## All you'll need: (makes 1)

2 tsp olive oil

½ small onion, thinly sliced

1 good-quality minute steak, fat trimmed

2 slices of sourdough bread

Handful of spinach leaves

1 gherkin, sliced

Salt and pepper

## Method:

1. Heat the oil in a frying pan over a low-medium heat, pop in the onion and fry for 5–10 minutes until soft and brown. Push to the side of the pan, ready for the steak.

2. Season the steak with salt and pepper and place in the hot pan. It needs literally 30 seconds on each side (unless you like your steak really well done, in which case give it an extra 15 seconds on each side).

3. Take the steak and onions off the heat while you toast the sourdough. Layer the spinach leaves and gherkin slices on top of one slice of toast.

4. Cut the steak into slices and use to top the spinach and gherkins, followed by the gorgeous onions. Cover with the remaining slice of toast, push down and slice in half. Get stuck in.

If you like mustard, it works really well with this sandwich – use it instead of butter or ready-made sauces.

# Yellow Coconut, Chilli & Lime Prawns

Golden turmeric powder coats the gorgeous prawns in goodness, while the coconut, chilli and lime bring the dish to life. This recipe works well with both prawns or chicken, and tastes just as good hot or cold, so it's super-convenient for busy bees happy to eat out of portable containers.

**All you'll need: (serves 2)**

160ml tinned coconut cream or full-fat coconut milk

½ tsp ground turmeric

½ tsp chilli powder (or to taste)

Juice of 1 lime, plus extra wedges to serve

250g king prawns (preferably uncooked), peeled

1 tsp coconut oil

1 red pepper, cut into strips

1 pouch of ready-cooked coconut or plain basmati rice

Handful of coriander, chopped

**Method:**

1. Pour the coconut cream or milk into a bowl, add the turmeric, chilli powder and lime juice and stir together.

2. Add the prawns to the bowl and leave to marinate for as long as possible (ideally overnight for maximum flavour).

3. Heat the coconut oil in a wok or non-stick pan and add the red pepper. Stir-fry for 5 minutes over a medium heat before adding the prawn mixture. Stir-fry for a further 5 minutes.

4. Meanwhile, pop the rice into the microwave to heat through.

5. Spoon the rice into bowls and arrange the prawn mixture around it. Garnish with the freshly chopped coriander and wedges of lime.

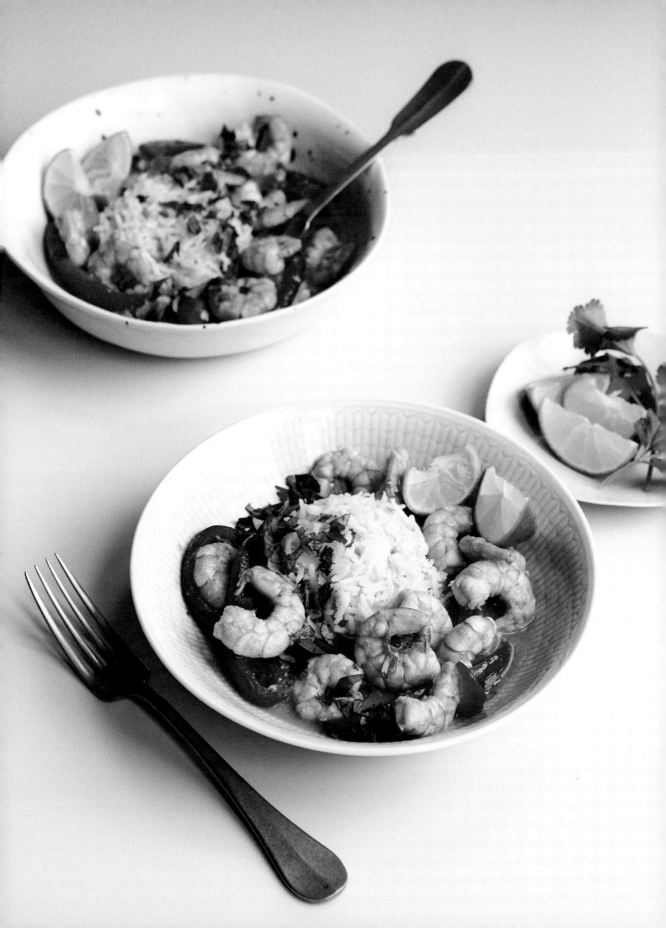

# Mackerel & Beetroot Salad with Horseradish Dressing

The sharpness of the pickled beetroot cuts perfectly through the sweet yet oily fish, and a spicy yoghurt dressing just tops it off. This was such a hit on my Instagram page that I had to include it here. Beetroot is a versatile veggie and one that I happily enjoy all year round, which is great because its health benefits are huge. Oily fish is packed full of healthy fats to help weight loss. It's a match made in heaven.

**GF**

**All you'll need: (serves 1)**

1 tbsp natural yoghurt

1 tsp horseradish sauce

1 lemon wedge

2 handfuls mixed salad leaves (watercress, lambs' lettuce, spinach, rocket)

4 golf ball-sized beetroots (I prefer pickled), cut into quarters

2 smoked mackerel fillets

4 walnuts, chopped

Salt and pepper

**Method:**

1. Mix the yoghurt and horseradish together, season with salt and pepper, add a squeeze of lemon and stir.

2. Scatter the beetroot over a bed of salad leaves, then flake over the mackerel fillets.

3. Dollop over the yoghurt and horseradish dressing, and finish with a sprinkle of crunchy walnuts . Tuck right in.

Feel free to swap the mackerel in this dish for tuna or any other healthy protein you enjoy.

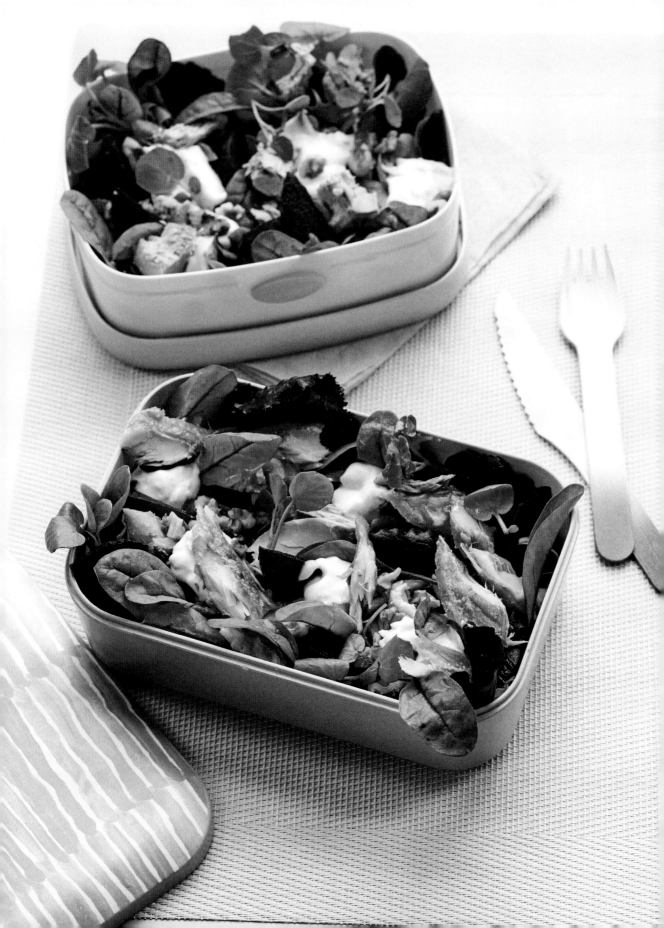

# Curried Cauliflower Soup with Poached Eggs & Soda Bread Rolls

This soup is flavoursome and warming, and the delicious soda bread rolls and protein-rich egg will keep you fuller for longer. The poached egg may seem strange to some, but honestly, the soft yolk gives the soup an amazing velvety finish.

## All you'll need:

### For the soup: (serves 4–6)

1 tbsp rapeseed oil

1 onion, chopped

1 large cauliflower (about 600g), leaves removed and florets roughly chopped

2 garlic cloves, finely chopped

1 heaped tbsp curry powder

400ml coconut milk or cream

500ml vegetable stock

4 free-range eggs

Salt and pepper

### For the soda bread rolls: (makes 8)

175g wholemeal flour, plus extra for dusting

½ tsp bicarbonate of soda

280ml buttermilk (or use milk mixed with 2 tbsp lemon juice)

2 tsp honey

2 tbsp pumpkin seeds (optional)

## Method:

1. Preheat the oven to 180°C/gas mark 4 and line a baking tray with baking paper.

2. First make the rolls. Mix the flour and bicarbonate of soda in a large bowl, then stir in the buttermilk, honey and 2 tablespoons of water. Bring together to form a dough, then knead gently. Tip onto a floured surface, roll into a sausage shape, then cut into 8 equal-sized pieces and form into rolls.

3. Place the rolls about 3cm apart on the tray, brush with water and sprinkle over the pumpkin seeds (if using). Bake in the oven for 20–25 minutes while you make the soup.

4. Heat the oil in a large pan, add the onion and let it soften and brown, about 5 minutes.

5. Add the cauliflower, garlic, curry powder, coconut milk or cream and vegetable stock and stir together. Cook until the cauliflower softens. Season with salt and pepper to taste.

6. Meanwhile, gently poach the eggs (see page 96); they add richness as well as some essential protein to the dish.

7. Blitz the cauliflower soup with a blender until smooth and creamy. Add more stock or water if you wish to have a thinner soup.

8. Pour the soup into bowls and top each with a poached egg and a final twist of black pepper. Serve with the soda bread rolls, using them to dip and capture all the flavours.

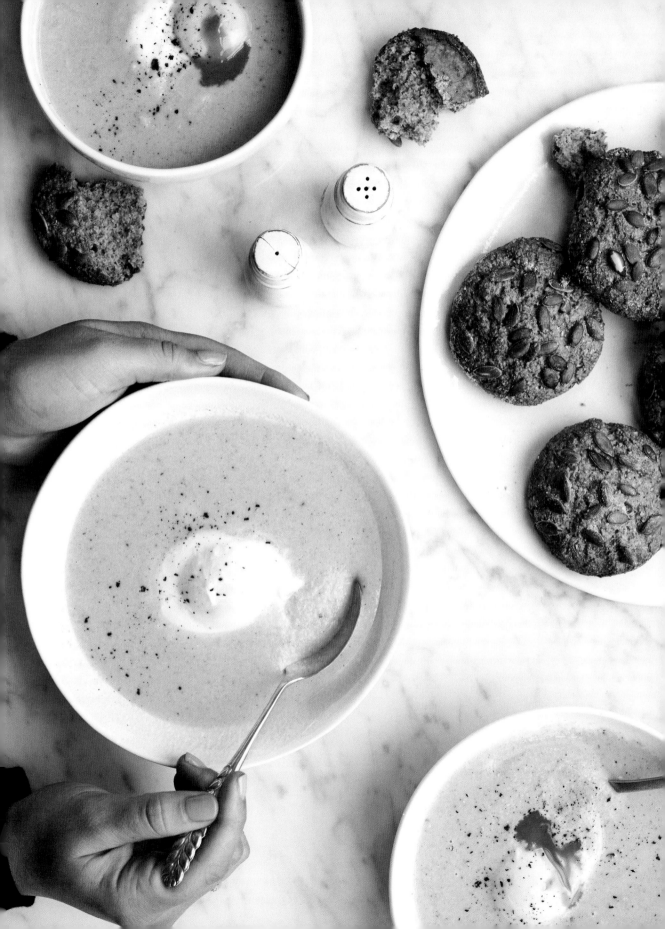

# Broccoli, Chicken & Cashew Nut Stir-Fry

This stir-fry dish is so simple and it can even be made in advance and heated up to suit you. I love the crunch of cashew nuts in this dish with the slight heat from the chilli and sweetness of the pineapple. So many stir-fry sauces are full of sugar and artificial colours and flavours with very little benefit to our health – it's time to start from scratch.

## All you'll need: (serves 2)

1 tbsp coconut oil or sesame oil

2 tbsp soy sauce

2 garlic cloves, very finely chopped

2 tsp cornflour (optional)

1 tbsp Chinese five-spice

Juice of 1 lime

4 skinless chicken thigh fillets, cubed

50g cashew nuts

160g tenderstem broccoli

80g buckwheat noodles

2 heaped tbsp chopped pineapple (tinned in its natural juices)

1 spring onion, finely chopped

1 red chilli, deseeded and chopped

## Method:

1. In a bowl mix the oil (you may have to melt the coconut oil first), soy sauce, garlic, cornflour, Chinese five-spice and lime juice.

2. Add the chicken cubes to the bowl and stir to coat, leaving them to marinate while you roast the cashews. To do this, add the cashew nuts to a wok or dry frying pan and place over a medium heat, shaking or turning them now and then to prevent burning until they go golden brown. Remove and set aside.

3. Add the broccoli and marinated chicken to the empty wok and stir-fry for 10 minutes. You might need to add a splash of water to prevent the mixture drying out and to help create a delicious sauce.

4. Meanwhile, cook the buckwheat noodles according to the packet instructions (usually 7–8 minutes simmering in boiling unsalted water).

5. Add the pineapple, spring onion and chilli to the wok and give the mixture another toss. After that, throw in the roasted cashew nuts. Finally, stir in the drained noodles so that everything is evenly coated.

# Super-Quick Pepper & Black Bean Chilli in a Jacket

You can't beat a jacket potato with a delicious filling. I try to keep my red meat consumption to just once or twice a week, so in between times I make this black bean chilli with Quorn, a vegan protein alternative which to me tastes amazing in dishes that are packed full of flavour and texture like this one.

**All you'll need: (serves 2)**

2 sweet potatoes (about 150g each)

1 tbsp oil

1 red onion, diced

300g Quorn mince

1 red pepper, deseeded and sliced

200g tinned black beans or kidney beans, rinsed and drained

1 x 400g tin chopped tomatoes

½ sachet of chilli con carne mix

Soured cream, to serve

**Method:**

1. Preheat the oven to 200°C/gas mark 6.

2. Pierce the sweet potatoes and pop them into the oven for 30–40 minutes (depending on size). You can also cook them in a microwave, but to me they taste so much better when baked in the oven.

3. When the potatoes have been in the oven for 25 minutes, add the oil to a pan and place over a medium heat. Add the onion and fry gently until softened. Stir in the rest of the ingredients and simmer for 7–10 minutes.

4. Remove the potatoes from the oven and cut down the middle. Fill each potato with half of the chilli and add a dollop of soured cream on top.

The chilli filling can be made in advance and simply reheated in the microwave at any time.

# Honey-Glazed Aubergine with Rocket & Goat's Cheese Salad

Salads don't have to be boring, and nor should they be. When I created this delicious salad, I found myself staring at an aubergine and thinking, what on earth can I make using you? Now this is one of my favourite go-to salads, and because you can have the aubergine warm or cold, it's delicious all year round.

### All you'll need: (serves 2)

1 aubergine, cut into cubes

1 tbsp rapeseed oil

1 tbsp honey

1 tbsp balsamic vinegar

1 x 200g packet of mixed salad leaves (rocket, watercress, spinach)

6 golf ball-sized pickled beetroot, quartered

6 walnuts, chopped

50g goat's cheese

Salt and pepper

### Method:

1. Preheat the oven to 180°C/gas mark 4.

2. Put the aubergine, oil, honey and vinegar into a bowl with a pinch of salt and pepper and toss so that the aubergine is fully glazed. Spread it out on a baking tray and pop into the oven for 15–25 minutes until caramelised.

3. Meanwhile, put the salad leaves, beetroot and walnuts in a bowl and toss together. Dot the goat's cheese over the top.

4. Once the aubergine is done, allow it to cool a little, then sprinkle it over the salad and enjoy.

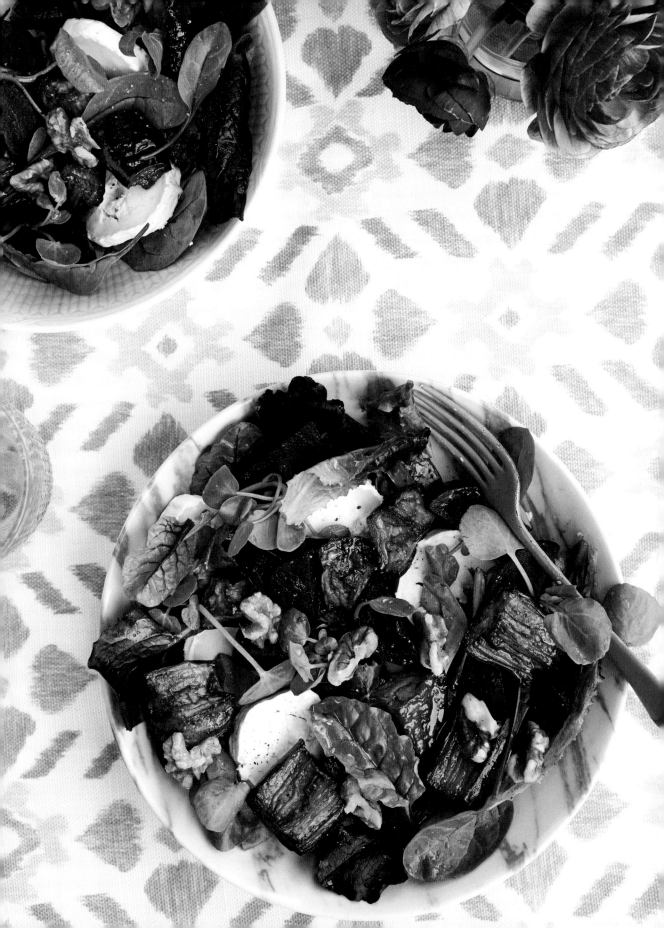

# Loaded Sweet Potato Skins

Think of an American-style restaurant chain where loaded potato skins are always on the menu. Crispy potato, salty bacon, tangy cheese and soured cream – what a dream! Well, here is my even dreamier version for you to enjoy; you may find yourself wondering why on earth you never had it before.

**All you'll need: (serves 2)**

2 large sweet potatoes

4 rashers of bacon, trimmed

2 spring onions, chopped

½ red pepper, diced

20g feta or goat's cheese, crumbled

2 heaped tsp soured cream

Paprika, to sprinkle (optional)

**Method:**

1. Preheat the oven to 200°C/gas mark 6.

2. Pierce the sweet potatoes and pop them into the oven for 45–60 minutes until soft. (You can also cook them in the microwave but you don't get the same caramelisation and crispness.)

3. While the potatoes are in the oven, place a non-stick frying pan over a medium heat and add the bacon, spring onions and red pepper. Cook until the bacon is browned and the pepper is soft. Meanwhile, preheat the grill to high.

4. Remove the sweet potatoes from the oven, gently cut in half lengthways, then scoop a good tablespoon of the flesh out of the centre. (You can save this for sweet potato mash, so it doesn't go to waste.)

5. Now fill each hollow with the filling you browned off earlier, sprinkle with the feta or goat's cheese and pop under the grill for a further 2–3 minutes. Add a dollop of soured cream and a pinch of paprika, if using, and get stuck in.

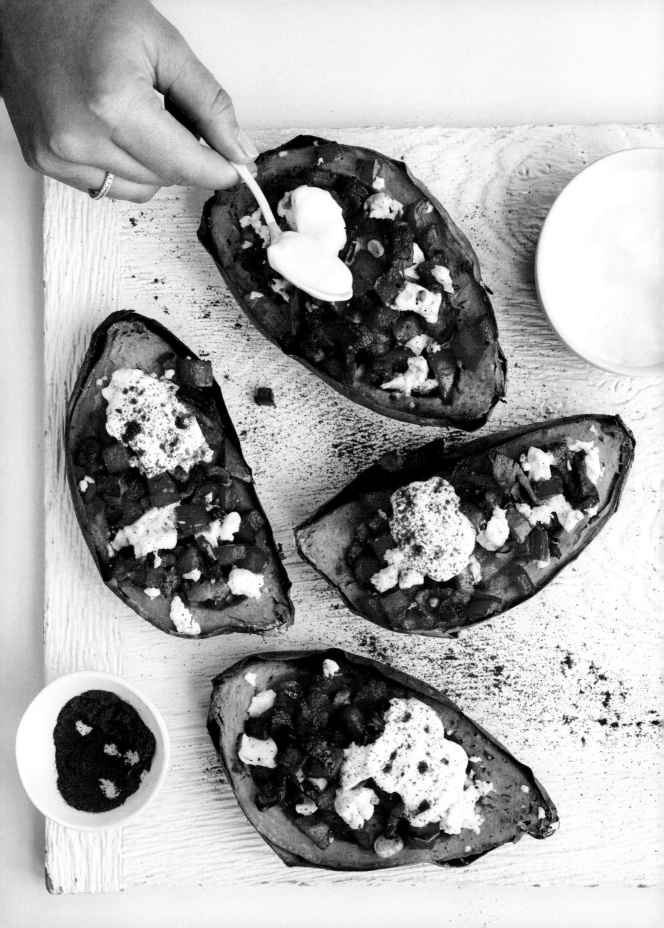

# Dinner

Dinner is my favourite meal of the day. I love comforting, heart-warming, family-style dinners that are easy to make but never fail on flavour. Ready-made sauces were such a common convenience when I was growing up, and still are for some people, but ditching them was one of the best things I did for my health and well-being. It forced me to learn about new flavours and was actually a real eye-opener to how convincing food packaging can be – light this, fat-free that . . . The truth is that once you have a good spice rack and the right store-cupboard staples, nothing is more convenient, healthy and rewarding than cooking from scratch.

# Spaghetti & Meatballs with Homemade Red Pepper Sauce

This heart-warming meatball dish is made with love. There are some days when I just crave pasta, and this is my go-to dish. It's quick and easy to make – in fact, the fresh sauce can be made while the spaghetti cooks. You won't look back.

## All you'll need: (serves 4)

120g spaghetti

1 courgette, spiralised or shaved into ribbons with a vegetable peeler

Parmesan shavings and fresh basil leaves, to garnish

### For the meatballs:

500g good-quality turkey mince or lean beef mince

1 large egg

2 spring onions, finely chopped

Salt and pepper

### For the sauce:

1 tbsp olive oil

1 onion, diced

1 red pepper, deseeded and diced

1 x 400g tin tomatoes

1 tbsp tomato purée

1 tbsp Worcestershire sauce

3 garlic cloves, crushed or grated

1 tsp chilli flakes

1 tbsp mixed herbs

## Method:

1. First make the meatballs: add all the meatball ingredients to a bowl and mix with clean hands until the mixture binds together. Divide into 12 equal pieces and roll into balls.

2. Bring a large pan of salted water to the boil and add the spaghetti. Cook for 10–12 minutes and keep an eye on it as you really don't want to overcook it.

3. Meanwhile, make the sauce: add the olive oil to a non-stick frying pan, pop in the meatballs along with the onion and red pepper and let them brown all over without cooking all the way through.

4. Once the meatballs are browned and the onion and pepper have softened, pour in the tinned tomatoes and tomato purée and stir. Let it simmer for 5 minutes. Add the rest of the ingredients, season with salt and pepper and simmer for a further 5 minutes.

5. Meanwhile, pop the courgetti into a bowl and heat in the microwave for 30 seconds to soften. Drain the pasta and combine the two together. This gives the impression of more pasta when actually you've got a lovely balance of pasta and vegetables.

6. Taste your pasta sauce to check you're happy with the seasoning. Then plate up and garnish with some shaved Parmesan and basil leaves.

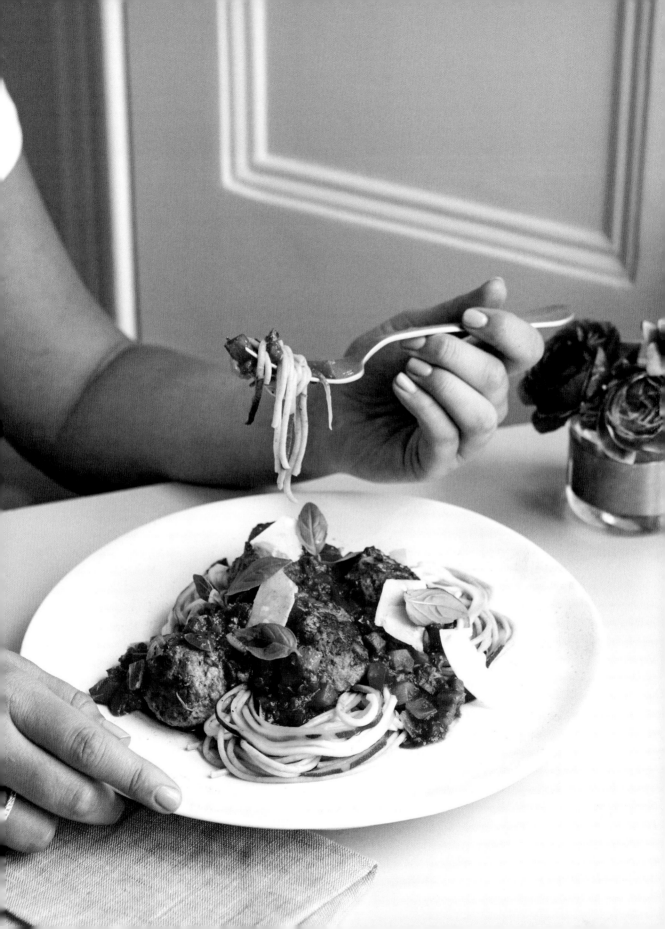

# One-Tray Roast Lemon Chicken with Honey-Glazed Veggies

There is nothing easier than putting a chicken in the oven; it does all the work for you. This dinner isn't just for Sundays, though; it's great during the week too, even if you're cooking for just one or two people. You can simply divide the chicken into quarters and save it for lunch or dinner over the next few days.

## All you'll need: (serves 4)

4 carrots, quartered lengthways

4 parsnips, quartered lengthways

2 tbsp honey

1 large free-range/organic/corn-fed chicken

1 lemon, halved

4 tbsp rapeseed oil

2 onions, roughly chopped into wedges

4 garlic cloves

12 new potatoes, halved

Sprig of fresh rosemary

Salt and pepper

Steamed broccoli, to serve

## Method:

1. Preheat the oven to 200°C/gas mark 6.

2. Put the carrots and parsnips into a bowl with the honey and some salt and pepper and toss to coat.

3. Place the chicken in the centre of a roasting tray and pop the lemon in the cavity (or you can roast it with the other vegetables) before rubbing some rapeseed oil onto the skin.

4. Surround the chicken with the onions, whole garlic cloves, potatoes, carrots and parsnips, mixing them around so they're randomly spread.

5. Drizzle some more oil over, season with salt and pepper and add the rosemary.

6. Pop in the oven to roast for 1–1½ hours, depending on the size of your chicken. With 10 minutes to go, make sure you prepare and steam your broccoli as a delicious side dish, and stir up some gravy if you fancy it.

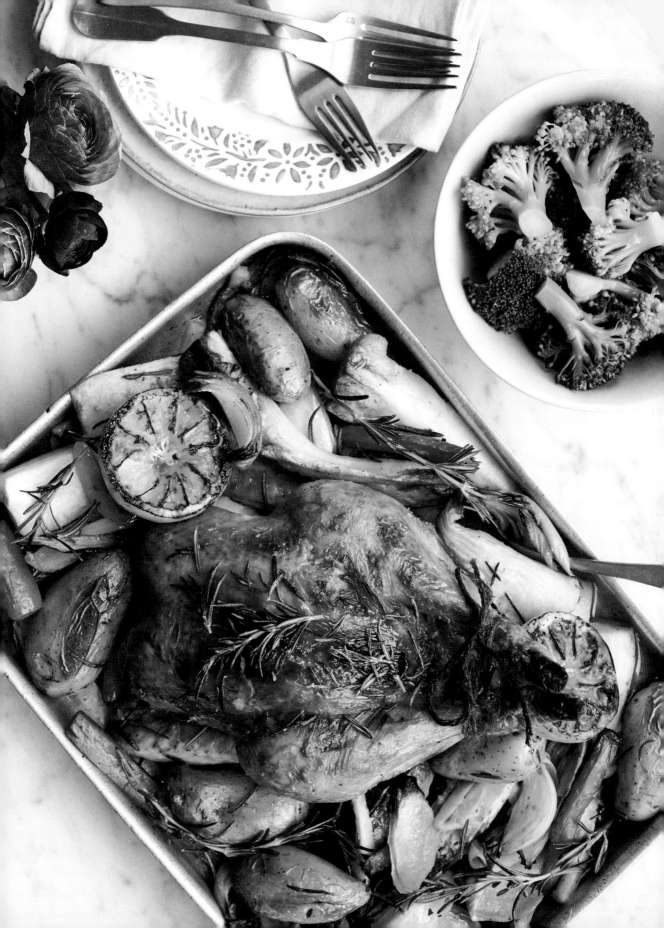

# Seared Tuna Steak with a Warm Asian-Style Sesame Salad

Fresh tuna steak can be pricey, but you'll often find it in the frozen food section for a great price and, honestly, it's just as good. Tuna is a super-meaty fish with an abundance of omega 3 fatty acids. It's lovely in this light dish, which is bursting with oriental flavours.

## All you'll need: (serves 2)

2 pak choi heads, leaves separated

150g edamame beans, fresh or frozen

1 x 200g packet of mangetout

2 tbsp sesame oil

2 tuna steaks

Thumb-sized piece of fresh ginger, peeled and grated

1 garlic clove, finely grated

1 large fresh red chilli, deseeded and chopped

2 tbsp low-salt soy sauce

Juice of ½ lime

1 tbsp sesame seeds (black and white)

## Method:

1. Put the pak choi, edamame and mangetout into a vegetable steamer (or into a colander placed over a pan half-filled with boiling water), pop on a lid and steam for 5 minutes.

2. While the veg steams, heat half the sesame oil in a non-stick pan over a medium-high heat. Add the tuna steaks and sear for no more than 2–3 minutes on one side.

3. Meanwhile, put the remaining tablespoon of sesame oil, the ginger, garlic, chilli, soy sauce and lime juice into a small bowl and stir until it becomes a lovely dressing.

4. Flip the tuna steaks over and sear the other side for 2–3 minutes.

5. Now remove the tuna steaks and set aside. Lower the heat under the frying pan, add the steamed green veg and pour over the dressing. Heat for a few minutes to warm up the dressing and gently coat the veg.

6. Tip the vegetables onto plates and top with the tuna steaks. Sprinkle over the sesame seeds and serve.

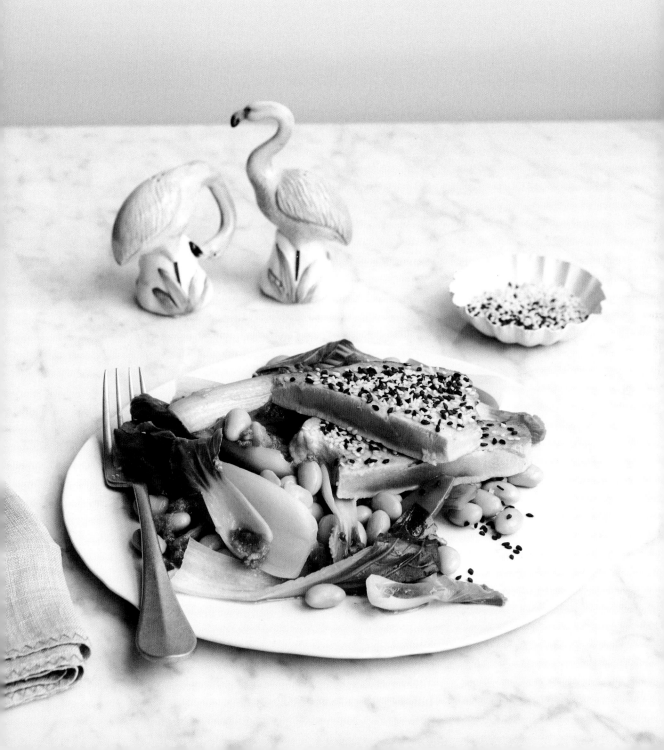

# Leek & Sausage Traybake with Sweet Potato Mash

This is simple, easy to make and a real crowd-pleaser. I recommend choosing very high-quality sausages that contain at least 90 per cent meat (unless you use veggie sausages, of course). You can get really delicious turkey or chicken sausages, which are the ideal alternative to pork.

### All you'll need: (serves 4)

8 high-quality low-fat sausages

2 leeks, cut into rough chunks

4 sweet potatoes, peeled and cut into rough chunks

Splash of milk

Knob of butter

1 tbsp gravy granules

200ml boiling water

Salt and pepper

### Method:

1. Preheat the oven to 200°C/gas mark 6.

2. Pile the sausages into an ovenproof dish and spread them out. Place in the centre of the oven for 30 minutes, adding the leeks after 15 minutes.

3. Meanwhile, bring a large pan of salted water to the boil and cook the sweet potato until soft.

4. Drain and return to the pan with the milk, butter, salt and pepper and mash until smooth.

5. Combine the gravy granules and boiling water in a jug; add more granules to thicken the gravy, or more water to thin it.

6. Remove the sausages and leeks from the oven and plate up on a bed of sweet potato mash. Offer the gravy separately.

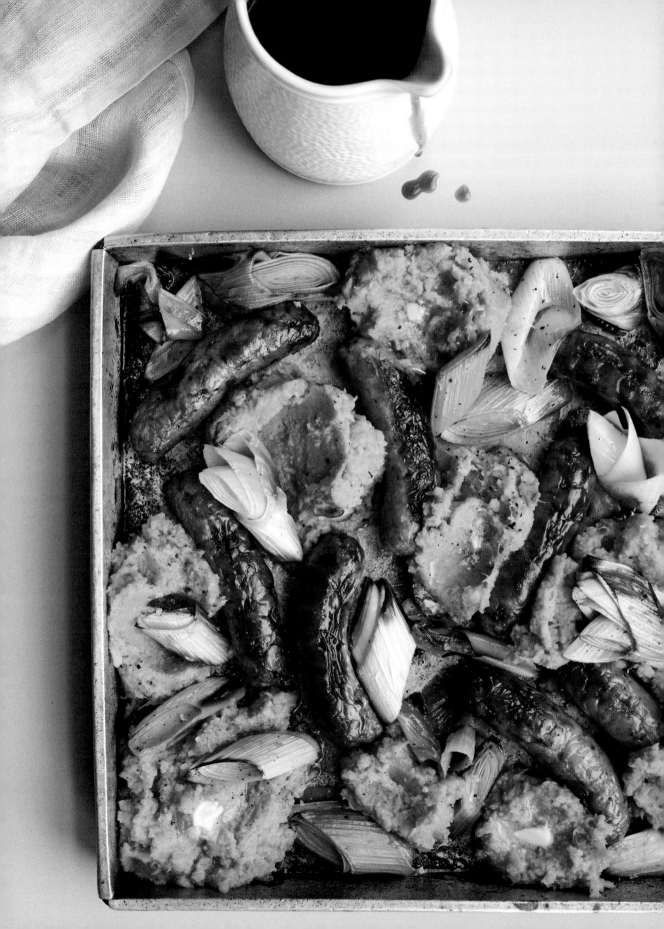

# Garlic Squash with Feta & Pomegranate Quinoa

Root vegetables are a great way to bulk up a dish while adding flavour and nutrients. Butternut squash is rich in antioxidants, potassium and vitamin A – perfect for keeping us healthy and glowing – so I've included it in this colourful vegetarian fusion of sweet pomegranate, salty feta and protein-rich quinoa.

## All you'll need: (serves 4)

1 butternut squash, peeled and cut into 3cm cubes

2 tbsp olive oil

2 garlic cloves, crushed or grated

1 tsp chilli flakes

400g quinoa

2 spring onions, chopped

4 tbsp pomegranate seeds

Juice of 1 lemon

100g feta cheese, crumbled

Small bunch of coriander, leaves chopped

Salt and pepper

## Method:

1. Preheat the oven to 200°C/gas mark 6.

2. Put the butternut squash in a bowl with 1 tablespoon of the olive oil, the garlic, chilli flakes and salt and pepper and stir to coat.

3. Spread out evenly on a baking tray (reserving the bowl of marinade for later) and roast for about 30 minutes until soft.

4. Meanwhile, rinse the quinoa in cold water, then tip into a pan, add twice the volume of boiling water and a pinch of salt. Boil for about 15 minutes, then drain.

5. Tip the drained quinoa into the reserved marinade, then add the remaining tablespoon of oil, the spring onions, pomegranate seeds and lemon juice. Season with salt and pepper.

6. Spread out the colourful quinoa mixture on a large serving plate and top it with the garlicky squash. Sprinkle over the gorgeous feta cheese and coriander leaves. Now everyone can get stuck in.

# Chinese Five-Spice Veggie 'Mince' with Fluffy Rice

This is a super-quick, stir-fry-style dish suitable for vegans, vegetarians and meat-eaters! Quorn mince is a great protein alternative as it is low in fat and high in fibre.

**All you'll need: (serves 4)**

1 tbsp sesame oil

1 garlic clove, chopped

Thumb-sized piece of fresh ginger, peeled and grated

1 red chilli, deseeded and chopped

2 spring onions, chopped

300g Quorn mince

2 tsp Chinese five-spice

2 tbsp soy sauce

**For the rice and broccoli:**

200g brown basmati rice

200g tenderstem broccoli

Drizzle of sesame oil

1 tsp sesame seeds

Pinch of chilli flakes

1 spring onion, finely chopped

**Method:**

1. First cook the rice. Bring a pan of water to the boil, add the rice and simmer gently for about 15 minutes without stirring.

2. In a separate pan, boil or steam the broccoli – your choice – until just tender.

3. When the rice has been cooking for 7 minutes, prepare the 'mince'. Heat the tablespoon of sesame oil in a wok, add the garlic, ginger, red chilli and spring onions and soften for a couple of minutes.

4. Add the Quorn, Chinese five-spice and soy sauce and stir or toss until the Quorn has softened – about 5 minutes as it cooks more quickly than meat. If the rice isn't cooked by this point, set the Quorn aside with a lid on to keep warm.

5. Once the rice and broccoli are cooked, drain the rice but quickly sit the colander containing it back over the empty pan and cover with a lid. This allows it to steam, which makes it fluffy.

6. Drizzle the broccoli with the sesame oil and sprinkle over the sesame seeds and chilli flakes.

7. Spoon the rice into bowls and top with the five-spice mince and sesame broccoli. Finish with a sprinkle of spring onion.

# Flaky Cod Parcels with Minted Pea Purée and Skinny Fries

Cod and peas with mint is such a fresh combination, and this recipe gives a little nod to our beloved fish and chips.

## All you'll need: (serves 2)

2 cod fillets (or use any white fish)

Lemon slices

2 sweet potatoes, cut into skinny chips (these cook more quickly than regular potatoes and go nice and crunchy)

200g frozen garden peas

50ml vegetable stock

Very small handful of mint leaves

1 tsp olive oil

1 tsp vinegar

Salt and pepper

## Method:

1. Preheat the oven to 180°C/gas mark 4.

2. Place each cod fillet on a sheet of foil and top with a few slices of lemon and some salt and pepper. Loosely fold up the foil to make two parcels, transfer to a baking sheet and bake on the middle shelf of the oven for about 20 minutes. Put the sweet potato skinny fries on a separate baking sheet and place in the oven at the same time, on the shelf above the cod parcels.

3. Meanwhile, pop the peas into a pan with the vegetable stock and mint leaves and bring to a simmer. Cook until the peas are tender, usually about 7 minutes.

4. Using a hand blender, blitz the peas and mint, then add the olive oil, vinegar and seasoning to taste.

5. Take the cod and sweet potato fries out of the oven, ensuring that the fries are nice and golden. Serve with the minted pea purée and more fresh lemon slices.

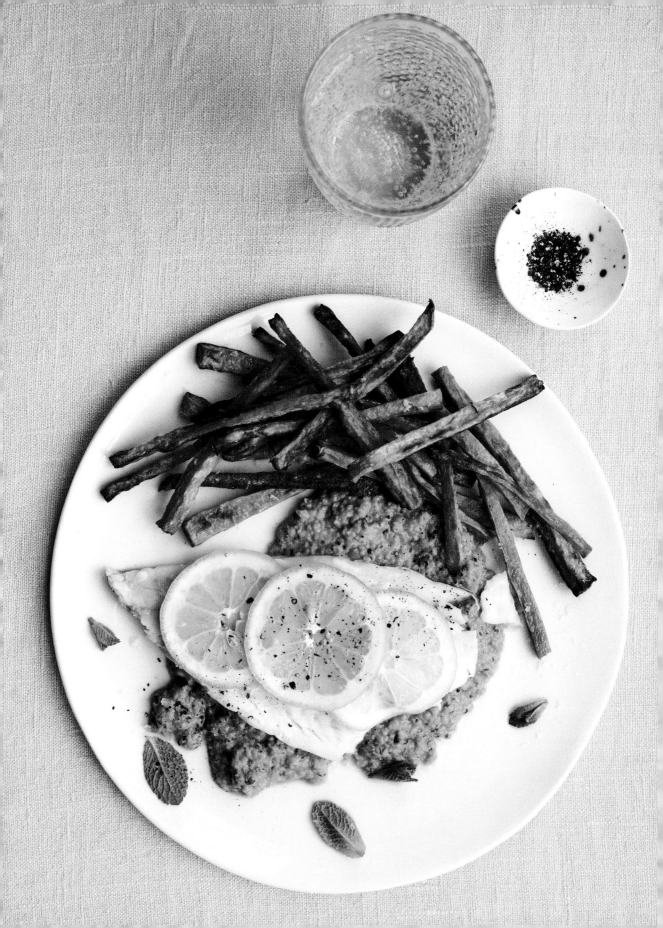

# One Pot Chickpea & Spinach Curry

This is great for those winter nights when you want to come home to a bowl of hot, filling food that just makes everything better. It's great for using up odd vegetables left in the fridge, and the long, slow cooking means it's ideal for making in advance. It tastes delicious the next day too.

**All you'll need: (serves 6)**

4 x 400g tins chickpeas, drained

1 large white potato, peeled and diced

1 x 400g tin chopped tomatoes

1 x 400ml tin coconut milk

2 red peppers, deseeded and sliced

2 heaped tbsp medium or hot curry powder

3 garlic cloves, finely grated

1 x 200g bag of spinach leaves

**Method:**

1. Put all the ingredients, except the spinach, into one large pan or slow cooker, then cover and cook over a low heat for 1 hour 20 minutes.

2. At the end of the cooking time, stir in the fresh spinach until wilted.

3. Serve the curry with a mango chutney and my Baked Onion Bhajis (see page 150).

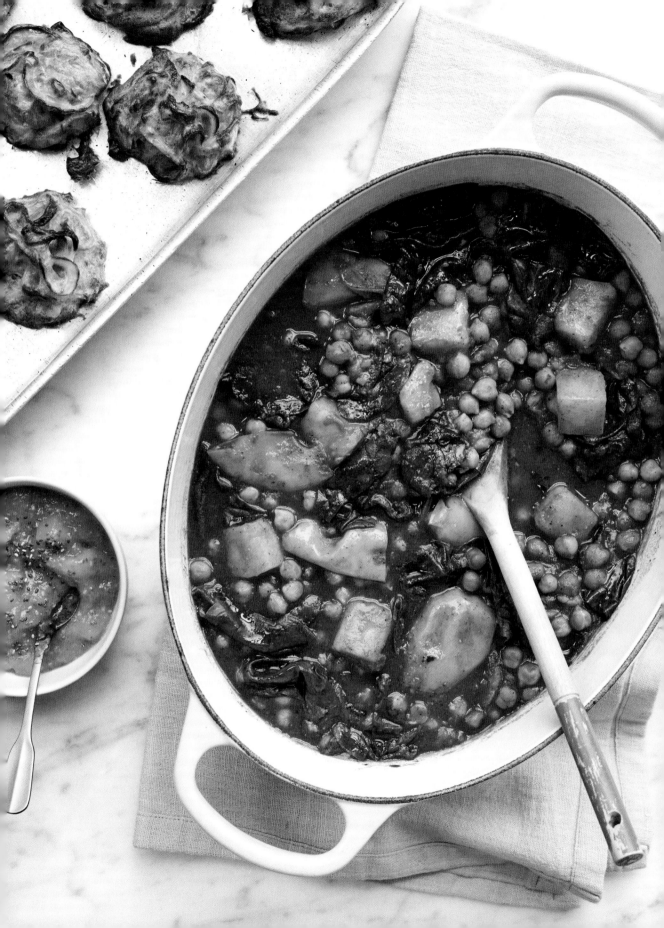

# Heart-warming Beef & Lentil Pie

Lentils are an amazing source of fibre but aren't always that appealing on their own, so I've added them to my beef pie. They work perfectly, giving the filling texture and added goodness.

**GF**

## All you'll need: (makes 4)

### For the filling:

1 tbsp coconut, rapeseed or olive oil

1 large white onion, finely chopped

500g lean beef mince

400g ready-cooked Puy lentils (I buy the pouches to save time)

250g frozen peas

500ml beef stock

Several splashes of Worcestershire sauce

2 garlic cloves, finely grated

1 tbsp cumin seeds

2 tbsp tomato purée

### For the topping:

½ swede, roughly chopped

3 carrots, roughly chopped

3 parsnips, roughly chopped

1 white potato, peeled and roughly chopped

Splash of oil or milk

Salt and pepper

## Method:

1. Preheat the oven to 180°C/gas mark 4. Set out four individual pie dishes, or use one large pie dish – whichever you prefer.

2. Put all the vegetables for the topping into a pan of boiling salted water and cook until tender, about 15 minutes.

3. Meanwhile, make the filling: heat the oil in a pan, add the onion and beef and stir over a medium heat until brown.

4. Add the lentils, peas and beef stock and stir again. Let it simmer and thicken for about 10 minutes.

5. Now add the Worcestershire sauce, garlic, cumin seeds and tomato purée. Continue to simmer for a further 10 minutes.

6. Once the topping vegetables are soft. Drain well, return them to the pan and begin mashing. Add some oil or a splash of milk to help bind them together and to get your mash as smooth as possible, then season with salt and pepper.

7. Spoon the filling into the pie dish(es), then top with dollops of the vegetable mash.

8. Now place in the oven for 10 minutes until bubbling and oozing (I love it when the gravy runs down the outside).

9. Serve with a side of greens, cabbage or sprouts.

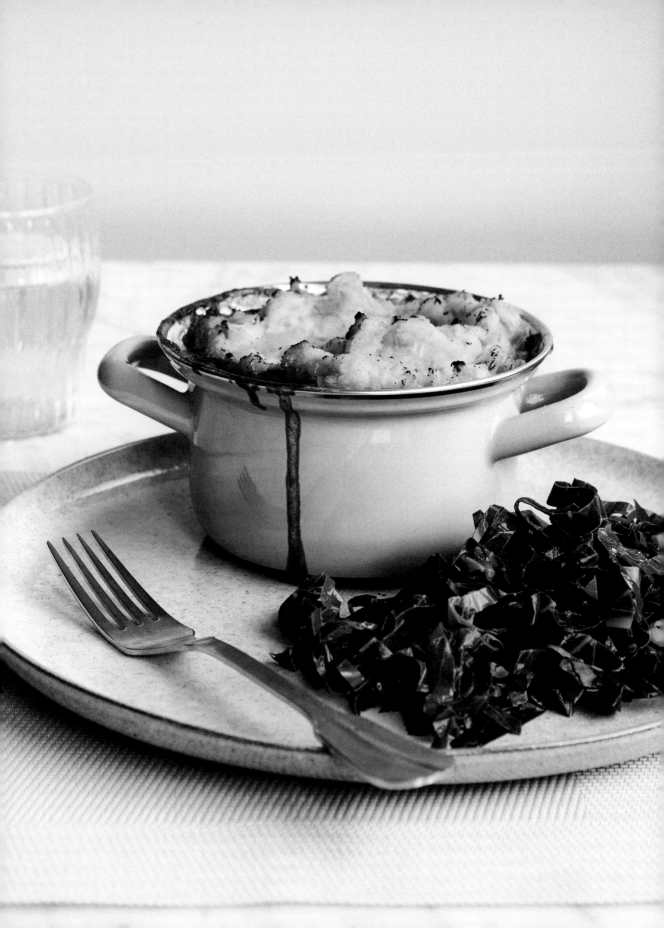

# Sticky & Spicy Drumsticks with Chunky Sweet Potatoes

Perfect summer barbecue food, these sticky and spicy chicken drumsticks are great with an array of salads, but can also be oven-baked in the winter with my chunky sweet potato cubes. Serve with yoghurt slaw, the ideal accompaniment.

**All you'll need: (serves 4)**

10–12 chicken drumsticks or thighs (skin removed)

2 tbsp sriracha (hot chilli sauce), or to taste

2 tbsp honey

1 tbsp coconut oil

1 tsp chilli flakes

Juice of 1 lime

4 garlic cloves, crushed

4 tbsp soy sauce

**For the sweet potato chunks:**

4 sweet potatoes, cut into 3cm cubes

Oil, for drizzling

Salt and pepper

**For the yoghurt slaw:**

2 heaped tbsp natural yoghurt

Juice of ½ lemon

1 tbsp salad cream

2 carrots, grated

½ white cabbage, finely sliced

Coriander leaves, to garnish

**Method:**

1. First marinate the chicken: put all the ingredients, except the chicken, into a large bowl and stir to combine. Add the drumsticks or thighs and stir to coat, then leave to marinate for as long as possible (ideally overnight).

2. Preheat the oven to 200°C/gas mark 6 and line two baking trays with foil.

3. Spread the sweet potato chunks evenly over one of the lined trays, season with salt and pepper and drizzle over some oil. Bake on the top shelf of the oven for 30 minutes.

4. Place a non-stick frying pan over a high heat and brown off the chicken drumsticks. Tip onto the second lined baking tray and pour over any remaining marinade for maximum flavour and no waste.

5. Pop the chicken into the oven to finish cooking for about 20 minutes.

6. Meanwhile, place the yoghurt slaw ingredients in a bowl and mix together.

7. Now pile the chicken, sweet potatoes and slaw on to separate serving platters and invite people to dig in.

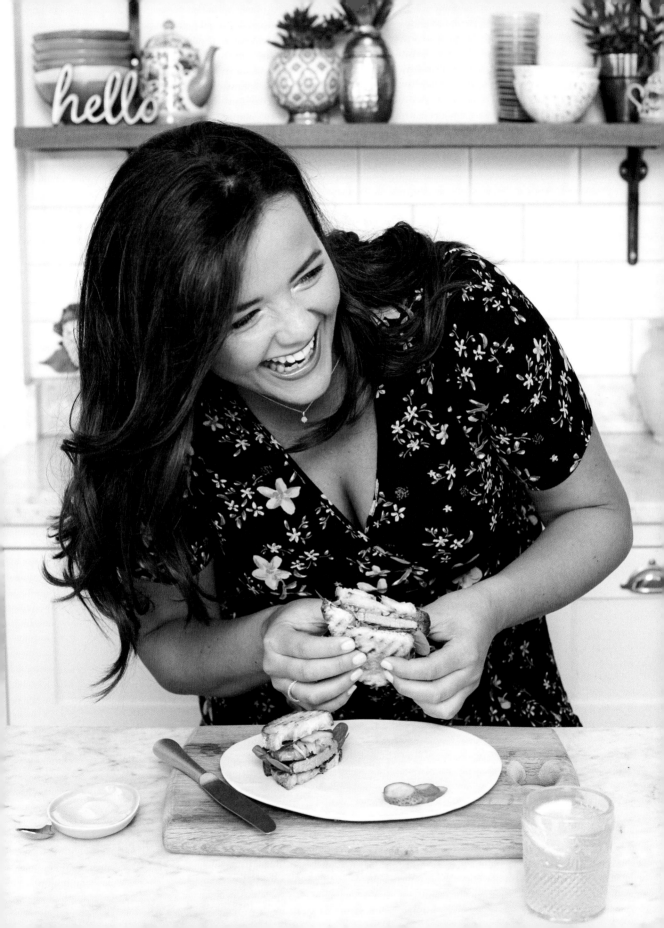

# Fakeaways

We all love a good takeaway; it saves us time and we can pretty much get any cuisine from around the world delivered to our door any day of the week. However, they are often quite greasy, cost a lot and we don't have any control over the ingredients used and the way they are cooked. If you love a cheeky takeaway a little too often, here are some recipes to give you the same flavours and delicious tastes with a lot more nutritional value.

# Kentucky Baked Chicken

Oh, we all adore that lovely Kentucky-style chicken, but deep-fried food on a regular basis just doesn't love us the same way back. This recipe can be made with chicken breasts, but I prefer it with thighs or drumsticks as the meat is a lot moister and it feels more like the real thing.

**GF**

### All you'll need: (serves 6)

60g rolled oats

1½ tbsp whole black peppercorns

1 tsp ground turmeric

1½ tsp garlic granules

2 big pinches of salt

1½ tsp ground paprika

2 eggs

12 skinless chicken thigh fillets

Drizzle of rapeseed oil or olive oil

### Method:

1. Preheat the oven to 180°C/gas mark 4.

2. Tip all the dry ingredients into a blender and blitz to a fine powder, then spread out in a shallow bowl.

3. Whisk the eggs in another shallow bowl. Now dip the chicken fillets one by one in the egg, then roll them in the powder. Make sure each chicken piece is generously coated.

4. Lay the pieces on a baking tray and drizzle over some oil.

5. Pop them in the oven and bake for 25–30 minutes, until the coating is crispy.

Serve this crispy chicken with some fresh corn on the cob and my Yoghurt Slaw (see page 144).

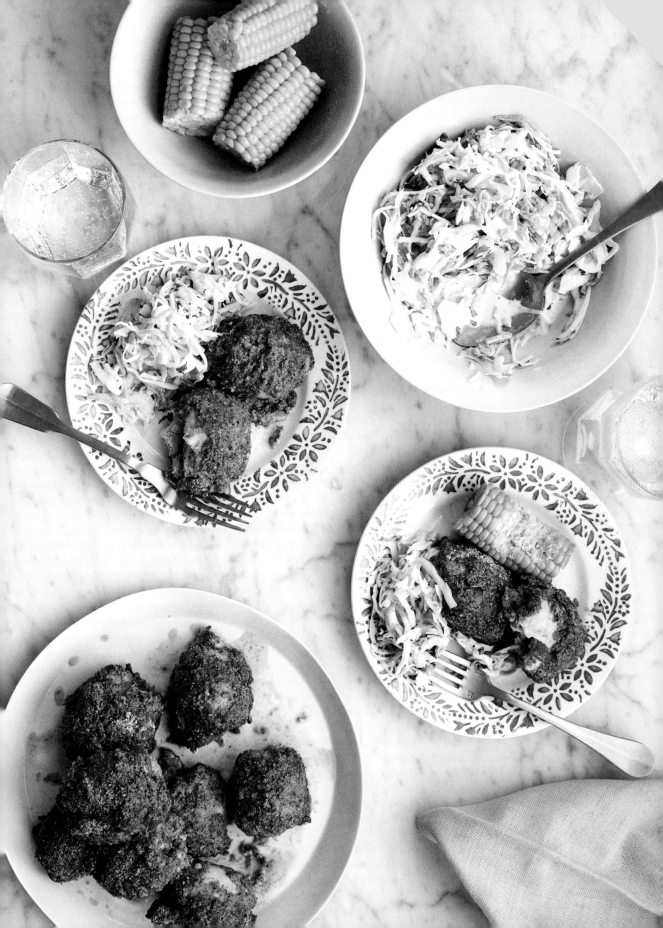

# Baked Onion Bhajis & Mango Jam

These crunchy, moreish bhajis are the perfect side dish to any homemade curry, but they wouldn't be the same without a mouth-watering mango dip.

## All you'll need: (makes 10–12)

### For the bhajis:

1 tsp rapeseed oil

3 white onions, thinly sliced into rings

2 eggs

100g plain flour (or use chickpea flour to make the dish gluten-free)

1 tsp ground cumin

1 tsp ground coriander

1 tsp ground turmeric

### For the mango jam:

225g fresh or defrosted mango chunks

Juice of 1 lime

1 tbsp honey

2 tbsp chia seeds

1 fresh red chilli, finely chopped

## Method:

1. Preheat the oven to 200°C/gas mark 6 and line a baking tray with greaseproof paper.

2. First make the jam: put the mango chunks into a pan and cook over a low heat for 5–10 minutes until softened. Tip into a blender with the lime juice and honey and blitz briefly so that the mixture still has some texture.

3. Tip into a bowl, stir in the chia seeds and red chilli, then set aside to thicken while you make the bhajis.

4. Heat the oil in a frying pan over a medium heat, add the onion rings and fry until translucent, then set them aside.

5. In a separate bowl beat the eggs and flour together with the spices. Tip in the onions and mix well (you might need to add some water if the mixture is too thick).

6. Now drop tablespoons of the mixture on to the lined baking tray, spacing the dollops about 2cm apart. Flatten slightly with the back of the spoon.

7. Once you've used up all the mixture, bake the bhajis for about 30 minutes until golden and crispy. Serve with the mango jam.

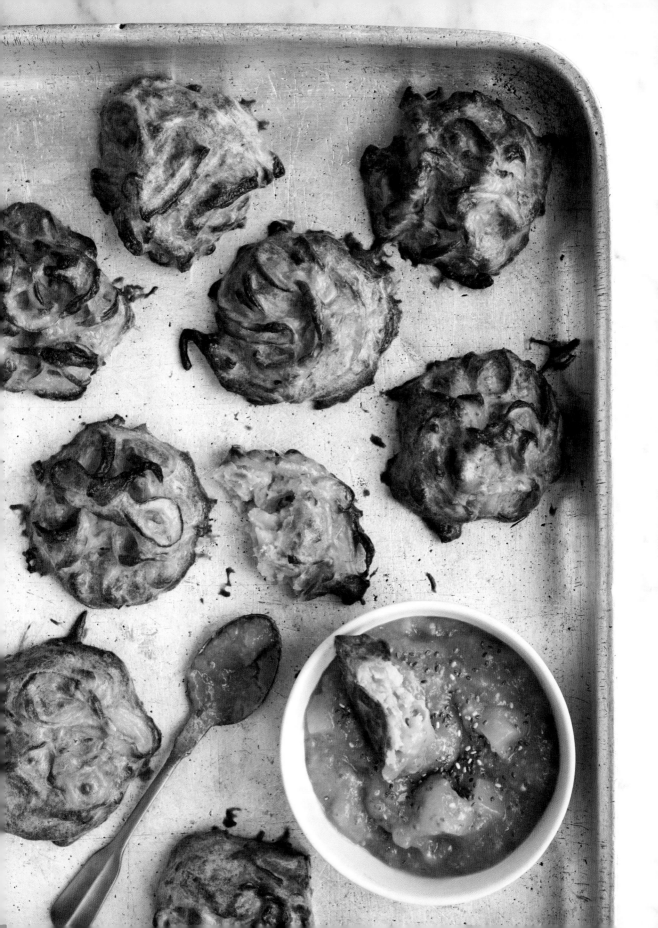

# Chicken Satay

A perennially popular dish in Indonesian restaurants, chicken satay is really easy to make at home. My satay sauce is also amazing with king prawns and a side of rice. Get the girls over and enjoy this with some delicious sugar-free cocktails (see pages 192–5).

## All you'll need: (serves 4)

4 tbsp crunchy peanut butter

2 garlic cloves, finely grated

1 tbsp mild curry powder

1 tsp ground turmeric

1 x 400ml tin coconut milk

1 tsp honey

1 tbsp soy sauce

500g skinless chicken breast, cut into strips

Handful of chopped peanuts

Handful of coriander leaves

2 spring onions, finely chopped

### To serve:

Basmati rice

Lime wedges

## Method:

1. In a large bowl mix the peanut butter, garlic, curry powder, turmeric, coconut milk, honey and soy sauce to make a delicious marinade.

2. Now pop the chicken strips into a sandwich bag and bash them flat with a rolling pin. Place them in the bowl of marinade and stir to coat. Set aside to marinate for as long as you can (ideally overnight).

3. Place a wok over a medium-high heat. Pour the chicken and all the marinade into the wok and cook, stirring, until the chicken is cooked through.

4. Top the satay chicken in the wok with chopped peanuts, fresh coriander leaves and spring onions. Bring the wok to the middle of the table and serve with basmati rice and lime wedges to squeeze over.

# Tasty Cheeseburger with Cajun Wedges & Garlic Dip

I often crave a burger, especially when I'm grumpy with hunger (perhaps I should say 'hangry'). There is something so satisfying about picking up a loaded burger with all the toppings, closing your eyes and taking a massive bite.

GF

**All you'll need: (makes 6)**

**For the burgers:**

500g turkey mince

1 heaped tsp ground turmeric

2 eggs, beaten

Oil, for brushing

6 thin slices of mature Cheddar

6 iceberg lettuce leaves (keep them whole)

1 beef tomato, sliced

12 slices jalapeño chilli

Salt and pepper

**For the Cajun wedges:**

3 large white potatoes, cut into wedges

Olive oil, for drizzling

2 tsp Cajun seasoning

**For the garlic dip:**

4 tbsp natural yoghurt

1 tsp garlic granules

Salt and pepper

**Method:**

1. Preheat the oven to 180°C/gas mark 4.

2. Spread the potato wedges out onto a baking tray, drizzle over some oil and sprinkle evenly with the Cajun seasoning. Bake for 30 minutes.

3. In a bowl mix together the turkey mince, turmeric and eggs and season with salt and pepper. Form into 6 equal patties, then place in the fridge for 10 minutes to help them keep their shape.

4. Brush a non-stick frying pan with oil and place over a medium-high heat. Add the patties to the pan and cook for 5–7 minutes on each side. Just before the burgers are cooked, pop a slice of cheese onto each burger so that it gently melts.

5. Stir together the garlic dip ingredients and set aside.

6. Now place each burger in a lettuce leaf and top with slices of tomato and jalapeño.

7. Remove the wedges from the oven and enjoy alongside the burgers and dip.

# Sizzling Thai Beef & Red Pepper Stir-Fry

This is a gorgeous fragrant dish that is best cooked with good-quality frying steak or rump steak. By making this yourself instead of opting for a takeaway, you'll be creating a delicious, healthy meal for two – something to feel proud of.

## All you'll need: (serves 2)

4 thin frying steaks

Flour, for dusting

1 tbsp coconut oil

1 red pepper, deseeded and sliced lengthways

1 red onion, sliced

50g green beans, trimmed

3 garlic cloves, roughly chopped

2 red chillies, deseeded and finely chopped

1 tsp oyster sauce

2 tsp soy sauce

1 tsp honey

10 Thai basil leaves

Salt and pepper

Rice noodles or coconut rice, to serve

## Method:

1. Cut the steaks against the grain into strips 2cm thick. Coat the strips with a sprinkle of flour and some salt and pepper.

2. Heat the coconut oil in a wok over a medium-high heat. Add the steak strips and stir-fry until browned, then add the red pepper, onion, green beans, garlic and chillies. Stir-fry for a few minutes until the vegetables soften slightly but still have a nice crunch to them.

3. Now add the oyster sauce, soy sauce and honey to the wok and let everything sizzle for a minute – just long enough for the flavours to combine.

4. Stir in the Thai basil leaves, and then serve with rice noodles or coconut rice.

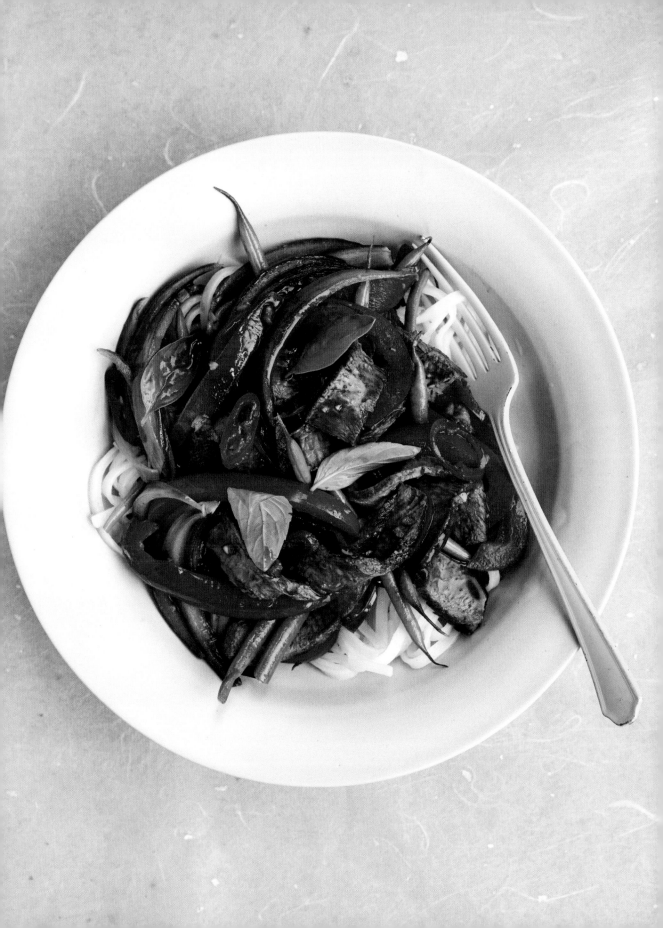

# Chocolate Cravings

Chocolate is my biggest weakness, and I often have a craving for it around that dreaded time of the month. Since I've been avoiding refined sugars, I find most milk chocolate is now far too sweet for me, so I often turn to a couple of squares of good-quality dark chocolate. If that doesn't hit the spot, I have some go-to chocolate heaven recipes that most definitely will.

# Chocolate Coconut Cups

My favourite chocolate bar was always Bounty, but now it's far too sweet for me, so I've made these delicious alternatives instead. If you love coconut and chocolate and need that hit of indulgence, keep these beauties in the fridge. They're free from refined sugar and just one of them most definitely hits the sweet spot to satisfy those cravings.

### All you'll need: (makes 9)

**For the chocolate bases:**

6 heaped tbsp coconut oil

5 tbsp cacao powder (not cocoa)

2–3 tbsp maple syrup or honey

**For the filling:**

75g desiccated coconut

3 tbsp coconut oil, melted

1 tbsp maple syrup

100ml coconut/almond milk

1 tbsp vanilla protein powder

### Method:

1. To make the bases, melt the coconut oil in a pan over a low heat and stir in the cacao powder and maple syrup or honey. As soon as the ingredients are combined, remove from the heat so that the mixture doesn't burn as this will make it very bitter.

2. Line a cupcake tin with 9 paper cases and spoon a level tablespoon of the chocolate mixture into each case (keep the remainder for the top of the cups). Freeze for 10–15 minutes, making sure the tin is level.

3. Mix all the filling ingredients together in a mixing bowl until combined and a sticky consistency forms.

4. Take the cupcake tin out of the freezer, top each frozen chocolate base with a heaped teaspoon of the coconut filling and press down or spread with the back of the spoon.

5. Pour a tablespoon of the reserved chocolate mixture over each cup. Freeze again for 15 minutes.

6. Let the coconut cups defrost slightly before serving.

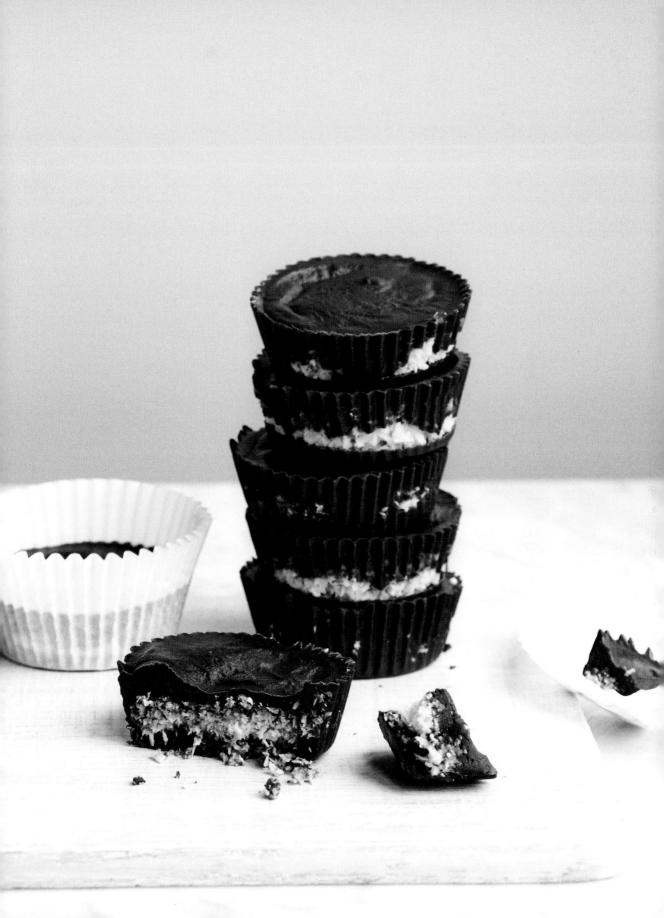

# Cherry & Hazelnut Chocolate Porridge

Think chocolate-hazelnut spread mixed with creamy oats and sweet cherries. This is my go-to breakfast when it's the first day of my period and I just crave chocolate and cuddles.

### All you'll need: (serves 1)

60g rolled oats

250ml hazelnut milk (or any nut milk), plus extra if needed

½ scoop of chocolate protein powder (optional, but a great addition that I'd strongly recommend)

1 tbsp chopped hazelnuts

6 cherries, stoned and halved

1 square of dark chocolate (at least 70% cocoa solids)

### Method:

1. Put the oats, milk and protein powder, if using, into a bowl and stir together, then pop into the microwave for 1 minute on a high setting. Stir again, adding a little more milk if necessary, and microwave for another 30 seconds.

2. Sprinkle over the hazelnuts and cherries and place the square of chocolate in the centre. Gently stir this in as it melts.

3. Sit down and close your eyes while you indulge in the yummiest ever bowl of porridge.

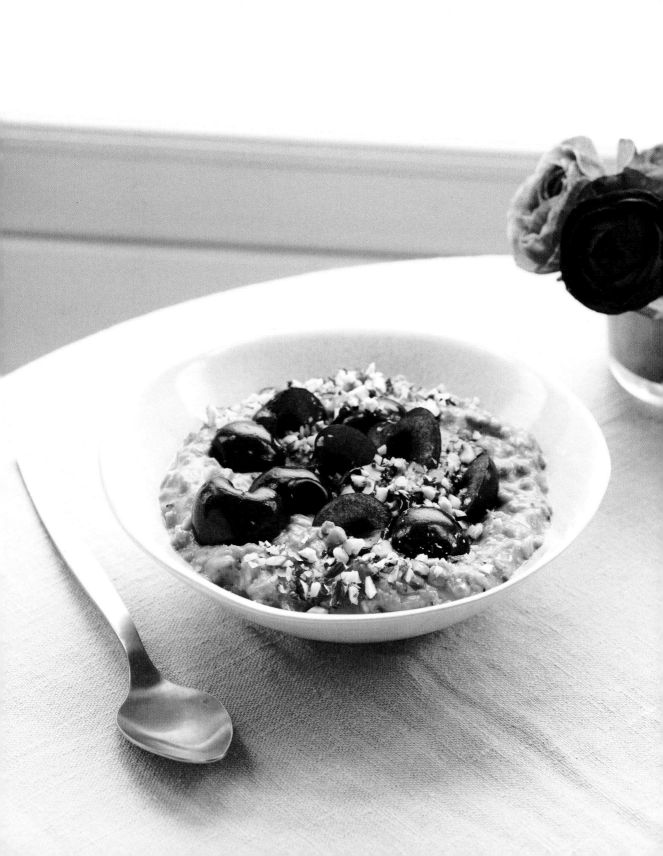

# Minty Chocolate Rice Crispy Bites

My mum used to make these at Easter time, minus the mint and with the addition of mini chocolate eggs for decoration. Rice crispy cakes are a classic. I recently found myself searching for something sweet, but the super-dark chocolate in the fridge wasn't enough this time. When I spotted the abandoned box of Rice Krispies staring at me, they finally found a purpose again.

All you'll need: (makes 12 mini bites)

100g dark chocolate (at least 70% cocoa solids)

1 tsp mint (or orange) extract

50g (about 2 mugs) puffed rice cereal

Method:

1. Place 12 mini cupcake cases on a plate or tray.

2. Put the dark chocolate in a large heatproof bowl and melt gently in the microwave. Check it every 10 seconds as it can easily burn.

3. Once the chocolate has melted, add the mint or orange extract, then stir in the puffed rice so it is completely coated.

4. Spoon into the mini cupcake cases and chill in the fridge for at least 4 hours.

5. Enjoy with a cup of tea.

# Chocolate, Chilli & Chia Layered Mousse

I think chilli and chocolate go so beautifully together that I decided to use them in a pudding-style chocolate treat that had a bit of a twist and felt a little luxurious too. Nothing is more indulgent than a chocolate mousse.

**All you'll need: (makes 4)**

4 pitted dates

4 tbsp chia seeds

1 x 400ml tin full-fat coconut milk

60g cacao powder (not cocoa)

1 tsp ground cinnamon

½ tsp chilli powder

4 tbsp maple syrup

**Extras:**

2 passion fruits

200g strawberries, hulled and chopped
   (reserve 4 whole strawberries for decoration)

**Method:**

1. Add all the mousse ingredients to a blender and blitz until smooth and creamy.

2. Halve the passion fruits and scoop the flesh into a bowl. Add the chopped strawberries and mix together. Place a tablespoon of the fruit in the bottom of 4 small round bowls or glasses.

3. Pour some chia mousse mixture into each glass, then place in the fridge for at least 4 hours to set.

4. Serve each mousse with a fresh strawberry on top.

# Protein Fruit & Nut Brownies

These fuss-free brownie bites contain no refined sugar and are great for providing a post-workout boost. They're also lovely with a cup of tea.

### All you'll need: (makes 9 squares)

3 ripe bananas (they don't have to be super-ripe, just a few dark spots)

2 tbsp chocolate protein powder

1 tbsp melted coconut oil

2 tbsp chopped dried fruit (apricots, dates, raisins, cranberries)

65g nut butter (look for varieties with no added sugar or salt)

30g cacao powder (not cocoa)

1 tbsp chopped nuts (hazelnuts, peanuts, almonds, pistachios)

### Method:

1. Preheat the oven to 160°C/gas mark 3 and line a deep 15cm square baking tin with baking paper.

2. Mash the bananas in bowl until smooth, then add the rest of the ingredients, except the nuts. Mix everything together, then tip into the lined baking tin and spread out evenly. The mixture should be about 5cm deep.

3. Sprinkle the nuts evenly over the top and bake in the oven for 15 minutes.

4. Let the mixture cool before cutting it into squares of super-delicious, nutty and gooey brownies.

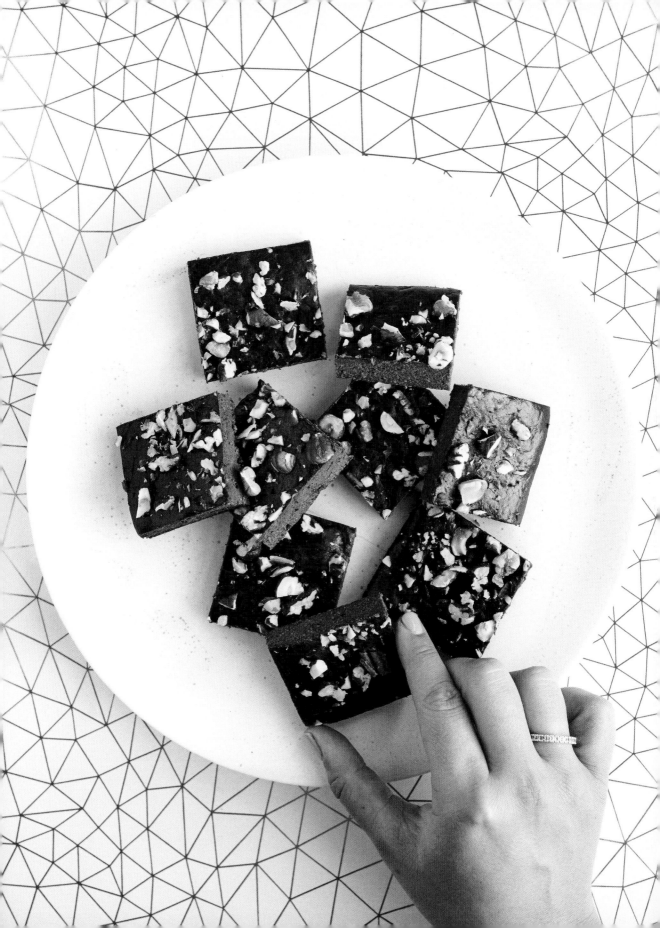

# Simple Snacks

Snacks shouldn't be complicated to make or require much cooking; they have to be easy to grab and go, giving you no reason to resort to shop-bought cereal bars or crisps. The recipes in this section are for my favourite sweet and savoury snacks.

# Strawberries & 'Cream'

A British summertime classic, this is wonderfully fresh and made in seconds. Strawberries are also packed full of vitamin C, and the natural yoghurt provides good bacteria for your tummy.

**All you'll need: (serves 1)**

6 large fresh strawberries, washed and halved

1 heaped tbsp Greek or full-fat natural yoghurt

A few seeds from a vanilla pod

**Method:**

1. Put the strawberries in a bowl, add a dollop of yoghurt and top with a few vanilla seeds for a super summery taste.

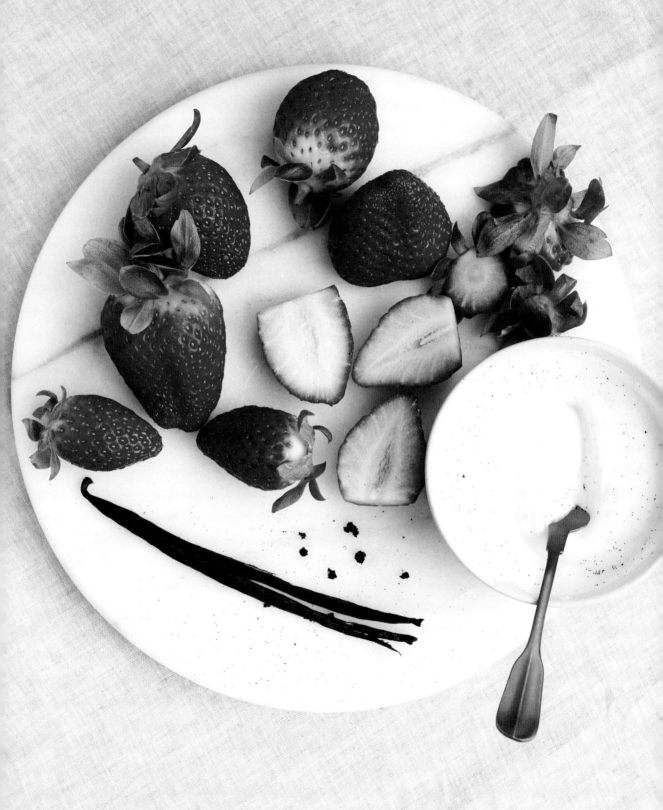

# Quick Mackerel Pâté with Cucumber Soldiers

GF

This is an ideal snack because you can make a nice little tub of the pâté and keep it in the fridge for several days, ready for instant snacking. If you decide to take it to work, make sure your container is airtight so that the fishy smell doesn't escape. Being oily, mackerel works really well with cucumber. Even people who aren't big fish-eaters love this pâté as the creaminess of the yoghurt mellows the fish taste so well.

## All you'll need: (serves 4–6)

280g smoked mackerel fillets (I like to leave the skin on as it's full of goodness, but feel free to remove it if you prefer)

2 heaped tbsp natural yoghurt

1 tsp whole black peppercorns

Juice of 1 lemon

1 small cucumber, cut into fingers

## Method:

1. Add all the ingredients, except the cucumber, to a blender and blitz until a smooth paste forms (you can have it coarser if you prefer, in which case blend for less time).

2. Spoon the pâté into a bowl or jar and scoop it up with your cucumber fingers.

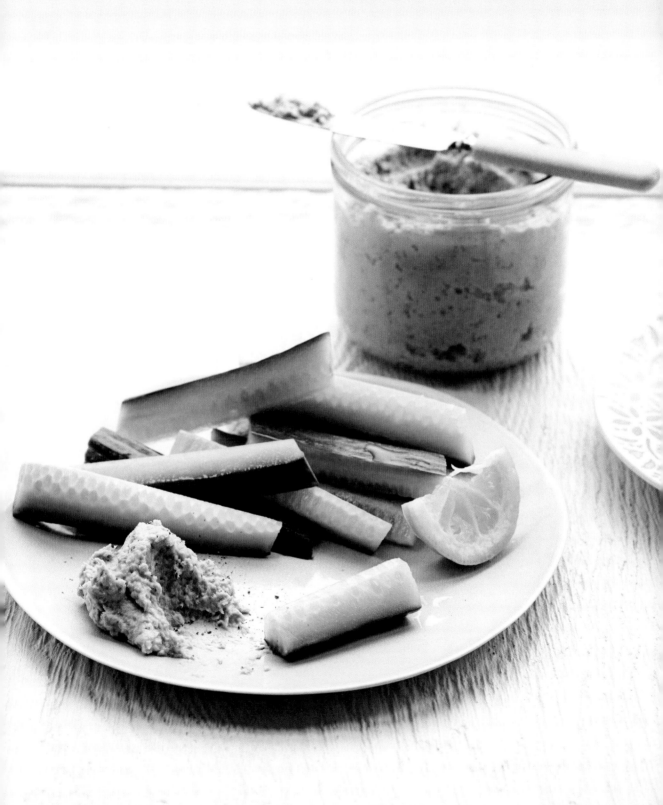

# Seasoned Crispy Kale Crisps

Even when I became aware that kale was one of the most nutritious vegetables out there, I still didn't eat it that much, unless it was in a smoothie. But then I discovered kale crisps, and couldn't believe how much the taste and texture were transformed. They are a great snack and a healthy alternative to potato crisps.

**All you'll need: (makes 2 portions )**

100g or 2 handfuls of kale

2 tsp olive oil

Juice of ½ lemon

2 tsp garlic powder

Salt and pepper

**Method:**

1. Preheat the oven to 140°C/gas mark 1.

2. Put all the ingredients into a bowl and mix together with your hands.

3. Spread the kale out evenly on a baking tray and place in the oven. Bake for about 10 minutes, but do keep an eye on it as kale can quite easily catch and burn.

# Peanut Butter & Banana Sandwiches

I love this little heavenly sandwich for a pre-workout energy boost; it's also a great 4 o'clock snack at work or at home.

**All you'll need: (makes 1)**

1 banana

1 tbsp good-quality nut butter (preferably peanut, as the flavour works so well)

**Method:**

1. Cut the banana into 4cm slices. Spread a small bit of nut butter on top of one slice and top this with another slice of banana to make a mini sandwich.

2. Continue sandwiching the remaining slices in the same way. You should get about 5–6 mini bites, which make eating a banana far more exciting!

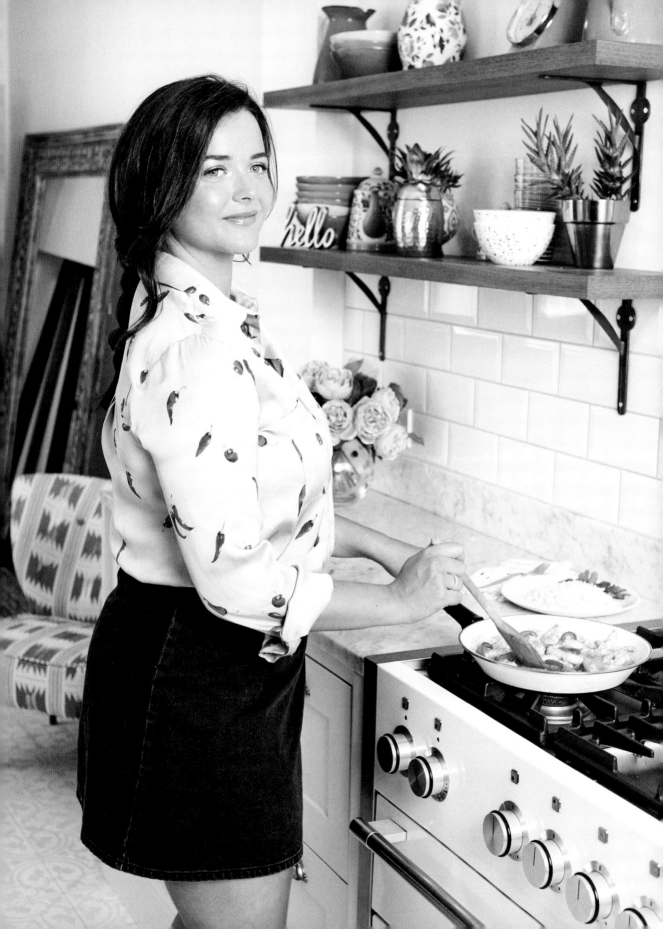

# Can't Be Arsed To Cook

This recipe chapter came from my most honest and realistic side.
I know and understand that some days we don't want to cook and
the idea of a ready meal or takeaway is so much more appealing.
Or maybe meal prep isn't for you (when I worked in an office it wasn't
always easy to organise proper meals).

For this reason I've put together some recipe ideas that
require zero cooking. Now please don't live off these meals; they are just
there for those days when you forget your packed lunch, or you've
had a series of late nights, or you just haven't
got the energy to cook.

# King Prawn Quinoa & Edamame with a Ginger Vinaigrette

Here's a simple but super-tasty salad to put together. You can actually get really delicious cooked prawns already marinated in herbs and spices. The coriander and garlic or chilli and garlic ones work amazingly well in this dish.

## All you'll need: (serves 2)

1 x 250g pouch ready-cooked quinoa

1 packet (about 200g) cooked prawns

1 x 175g tub ready-cooked edamame beans
(these are usually in the salad section)

### For the dressing:

4 tbsp sesame oil

½ tsp ground ginger

1 tbsp balsamic vinegar

## Method:

1. Pop the quinoa pouch in the microwave to heat up, following the instructions on the packet.

2. Put the prawns, edamame and quinoa in a bowl and mix together.

3. Combine the dressing ingredients in a cup or jug, stir well and pour over the salad.

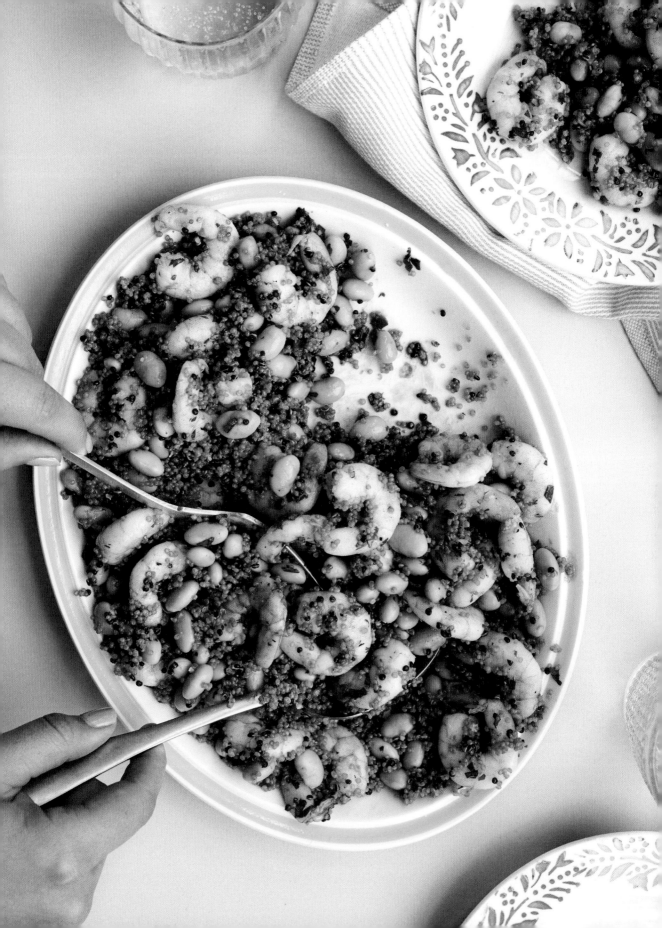

# Poached Salmon Fillet with Mixed Beans & Avocado

It's usually possible to find tubs of mixed beans in the salad section of supermarkets, and some even include avocado. If not, check out the tinned beans or the mixtures sold in pouches. Add some chopped avocado and you've got a gorgeous Mexican - inspired salmon dish.

**All you'll need: (serves 2)**

1 x 175g tub mixed bean salad

1 ripe avocado, peeled and chopped

2 tbsp tinned sweetcorn (no added sugar)

Handful of spinach leaves

1 poached salmon fillet (look in the chiller cabinets near the cooked meat and fish)

**Method:**

1. Tip the beans into a bowl, rinsing and draining them first if tinned. Gently stir in the avocado and sweetcorn.

2. Arrange the spinach leaves on a plate and spoon the bean mixture over them. Flake the salmon fillet into chunks and sprinkle on top.

# Classic Tuna Bloomer

I'm not a fan of supermarket sandwiches. After realising how much mayonnaise and salt they contained, I was quite put off. It actually works out a lot better value for money if you whip up your own and, most importantly, it's a lot healthier.

## All you'll need: (makes 1)

1 x 80g tin tuna in spring water, drained

1 spring onion, very finely chopped

2 heaped tsp mayonnaise

Black pepper

2 slices of fresh granary/seeded bloomer

4 slices of tomato, deseeded

4 slices of cucumber

4 thin slices of avocado

## Method:

1. In a bowl mix the tuna, spring onion and mayonnaise with plenty of black pepper.

2. Spread the mixture onto 1 slice of bread, then layer the salad ingredients on top.

3. Top with the remaining slice of bread, cut in half and enjoy.

# Ricotta, Avocado & Tomato on Rye with a Pesto Drizzle

This is a gorgeous open sandwich. When rye bread is toasted, it has a lovely honey flavour, which is delicious when topped with creamy ricotta, avocado and sweet cherry tomatoes.

## All you'll need: (makes 1)

2 slices of rye bread

50g ricotta cheese

½ avocado, sliced

10 mixed tomatoes, chopped (I like to use yellow and red or plum tomatoes)

### For the pesto drizzle:

1 tbsp pine nuts

Small handful of basil leaves

3 tbsp olive oil

Pinch of salt

## Method:

1. Blitz the pesto ingredients together in a blender.

2. Pop the rye bread in the toaster. When done, spread the ricotta on each slice. Layer the avocado and tomatoes on top.

3. Lastly, drizzle over the pesto and enjoy!

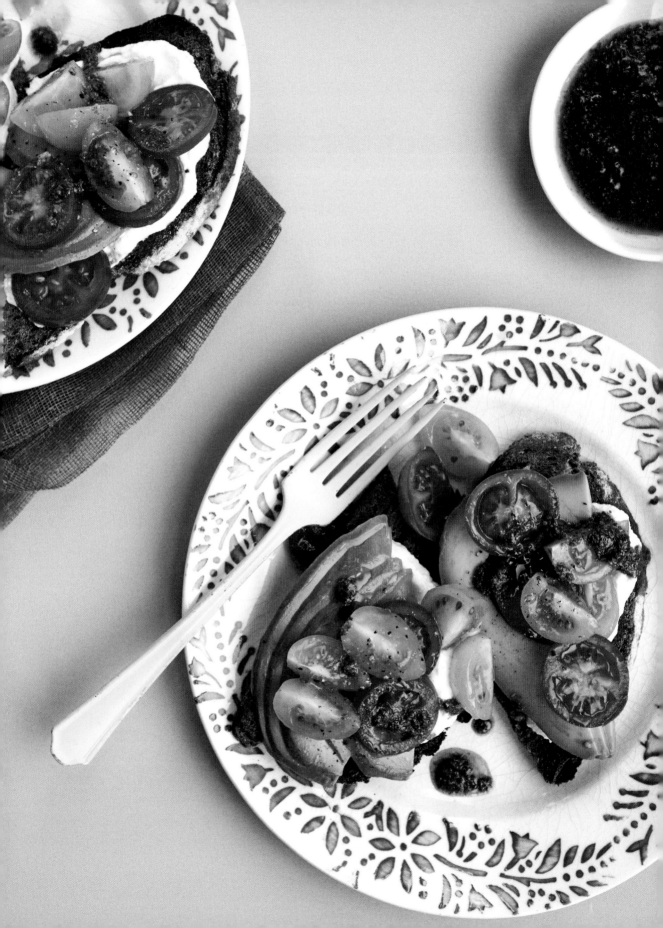

# Greek-Style Chicken & Houmous Wraps

All you'll need to take this chicken wrap to the next level is a microwave. Warm chicken and houmous in a wrap ... what's not to love?

## All you'll need: (makes 1)

½ packet (about 50g) cooked chicken slices (preferably harissa- or Cajun-flavoured)

1 tbsp houmous

1 wholemeal wrap

Handful of lettuce leaves

2 slices of tomato

4 slices of cucumber

1 tbsp crumbled feta cheese

## Method:

1. Put the chicken on a plate and pop into the microwave for 20 seconds on a high setting to warm up.

2. Now put the wrap in the microwave for 30 seconds on a low setting to warm up (it also becomes more flexible).

3. Spread the houmous onto the wrap and lay the chicken in a line down the centre. Top with the lettuce leaves, tomatoes, cucumber and feta.

4. Roll it up and enjoy.

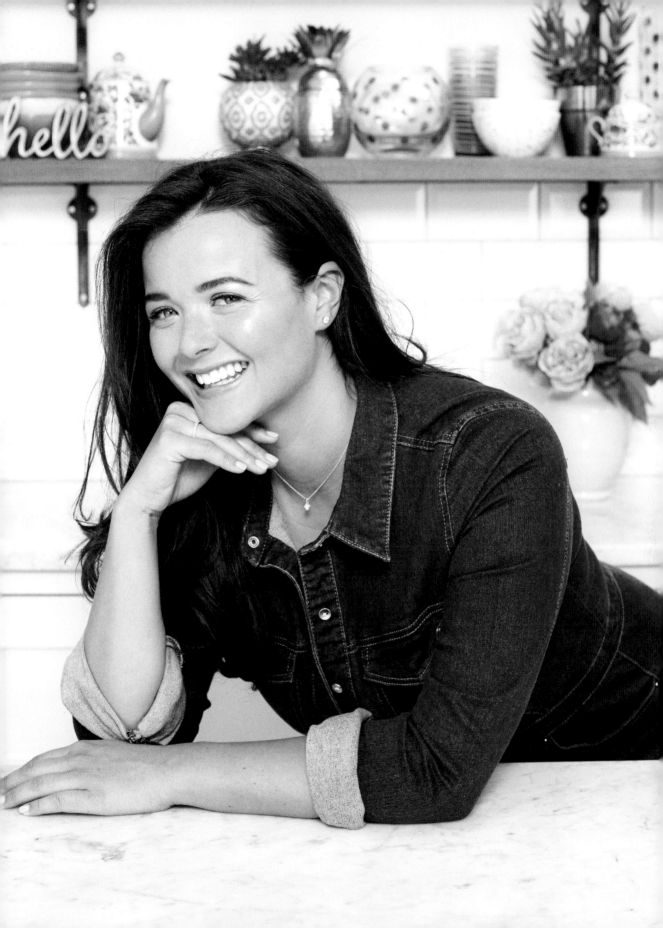

# Smoothies & Shakes

It's so important to get enough fruit and vegetables in your daily diet. They provide essential vitamins and minerals needed by the body in order to function effectively. Smoothies are a great way of consuming these things; they're also handy for using up leftover fruits and veg, which cuts down on waste. I prefer to have smoothies that are 70 per cent vegetables and herbs and 30 per cent fruits to balance out sugar levels.

# My Very Berry Smoothie

Berries are full of vitamin C, while spinach is full of iron, making this a delicious energy - boosting smoothie.

**All you'll need: (serves 1)**

150g mixed frozen berries

1 heaped tbsp Greek yoghurt

Handful of spinach leaves

100ml water

**Method:**

1. Put all the ingredients in a blender and blitz together until smooth and creamy.

2. Pour into a glass and drink straight away.

# Pine & Ginger Smoothie

A gorgeous tropical - inspired smoothie, this works well with a scoop of protein powder too. The oats make it quite filling, but it works perfectly with a light brunch.

**All you'll need: (serves 1)**

100ml coconut water

2 ice cubes

2 sticks of fresh pineapple

Thumb-sized piece of fresh ginger, peeled

1 tbsp rolled oats

1 tbsp natural yoghurt (use Greek if you like)

**Method:**

1. Put all the ingredients in a blender and blitz together until nice and creamy.

2. Pour into a glass and drink straight away.

# Super Green Smoothie

It's not always easy to eat all the fruits and vegetables required for maximum nutrients in their whole form. At the same time, some people worry that green smoothies might not be to their taste. Believe me, with the right ingredients they can be really refreshing!

**All you'll need: (serves 1)**

Handful of kale

Juice of 1 lime

½ avocado

8cm piece of cucumber

1 green apple

Cube of fresh ginger, peeled

100ml water

2 ice cubes

**Method:**

1. Put all the ingredients in a blender and blitz together until smooth. Add more water for a thinner consistency.

2. Pour into a glass and drink straight away.

# Vanilla Strawberry Shake

Keep it super-simple with this shake, which is ideal post-workout. Fresh fruit replenishes lost sugars, while that all-important protein sees to muscle repair.

**All you'll need: (makes 1)**

1 scoop of vanilla protein powder

5 strawberries

½ banana

200ml nut milk

4 ice cubes

½ tsp vanilla extract

**Method:**

1. Put all the ingredients in a blender and blitz together until creamy.

2. Pour into a glass and drink straight away.

# Cacao Coffee Shake

I absolutely love this shake in the mornings, as it has that coffee kick. If I'm in a hurry, I'll whizz this up and add a scoop of rolled oats to keep me full until early lunchtime. It also works perfectly as an iced coffee in the summer months.

**All you'll need: (makes 1)**

1 scoop of chocolate protein powder

1 tsp instant coffee granules, dissolved in a splash of hot water

200ml nut milk

1 tsp cacao powder (not cocoa)

½ banana

4 ice cubes

**Method:**

1. Put all the ingredients in a blender and blitz together until thick and frothy. Add extra ice for that yummy iced coffee taste.

2. Pour into a glass and drink straight away.

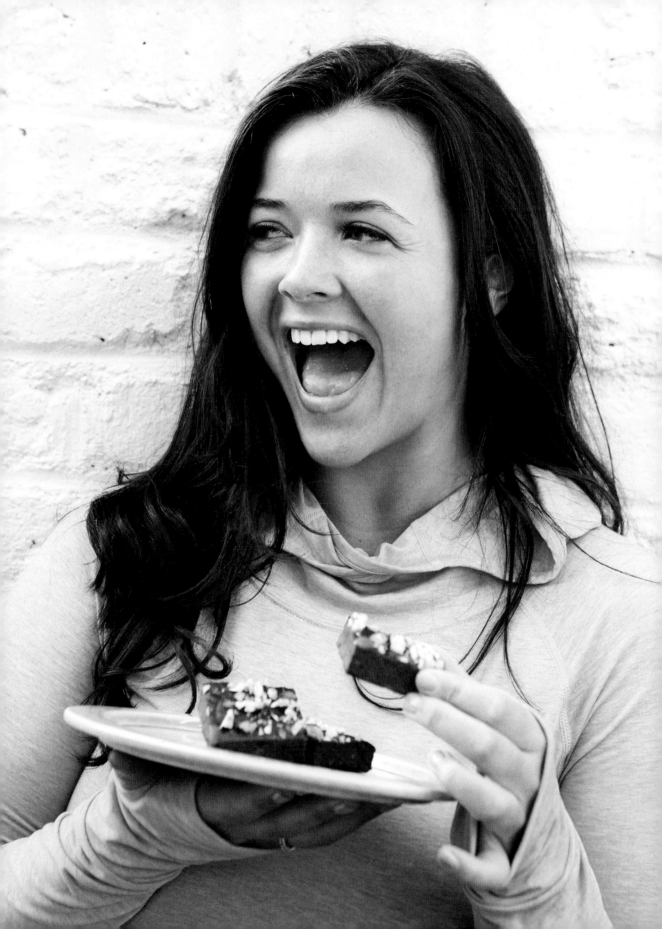

# Cocktails

Remember, *Healthy Forever* is about being able to live your life to the fullest from a health perspective while at the same time being realistic and still enjoying yourself. Making cocktails and cooking for friends is something I love to do, so maybe you can give it a go too? The cocktail recipes have been created to avoid refined sugars, and I've named them after some of my gorgeous friends.

# Connie's Vanilla Sour

This is my jazzed-up version of the classic vodka, soda and fresh lime. Sometimes you just need that extra burst of flavour.

**Serving suggestion:** in a tall highball glass with lots of ice

**All you'll need: (serves 1)**

4 ice cubes

1 measure (25ml) of vanilla vodka

¼ tsp vanilla bean paste or extract (optional)

Juice of ½ lime

Juice of ½ lemon

Soda water

**Method:**

1. Pop the ice cubes into a glass, followed by the vodka, vanilla bean paste or extract and the lime and lemon juices.

2. Top up with the soda water and stir.

# Debbie's Strawberry Crush

Debbie doesn't like too much fruit juice in her cocktails, which isn't a bad thing as fruit juice can contain a lot of sugar, so I make this Strawberry Crush for when she comes round. It's still really fruity and packed full of that genuine strawberry flavour.

**Serving suggestion:** in a fancy cocktail glass

**All you'll need: (serves 1)**

1 measure (25ml) of white rum

3 juicy ripe strawberries

100ml cranberry juice (no added sugar)

6 ice cubes

Juice of ½ lime

**Method:**

1. Put all the ingredients, except the lime juice, into a blender and blitz until slushy but not completely liquid – you still want that crushed ice texture.

2. Pour into a fancy cocktail glass, squeeze in the lime juice and enjoy. (If you want to make it fizzy, feel free to top it up with soda water.)

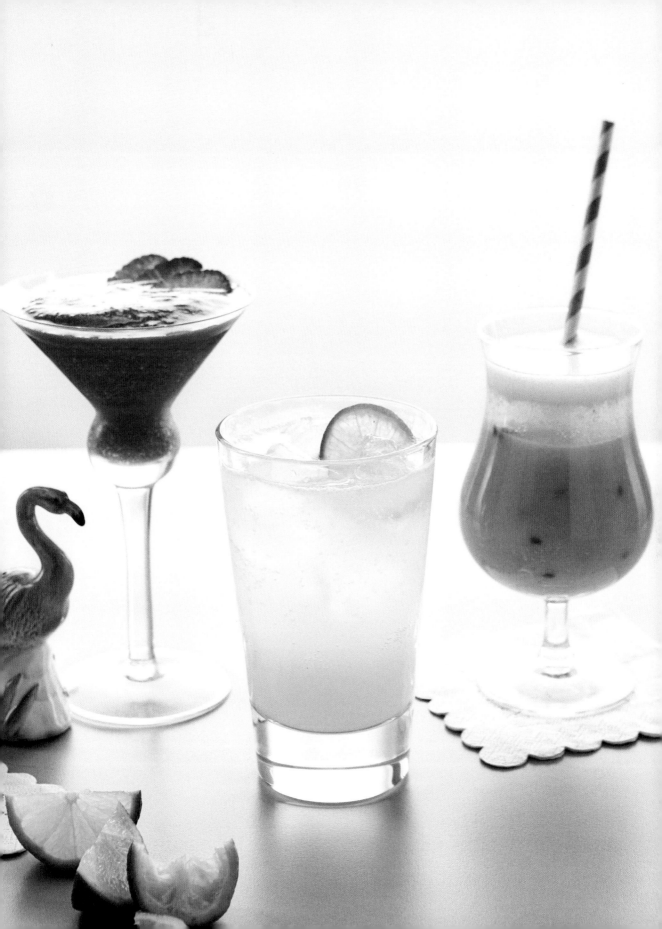

# Tara's Passion Fruit Mango Martini

This is a twist on a very popular classic that Tara loves. It's sharp, sweet and finished off with a shot of bubbles. It's perfect for anyone who loves tropical flavours but doesn't like missing out on a glass of bubbly. Here you get the best of both!

**Serving suggestion:** in a fancy martini glass

All you'll need: (serves 1)

4 ice cubes

150ml water or sugar-free tropical juice

75g freshly chopped mango

1 measure (25ml) of vanilla vodka

Juice of ½ lime

Passion fruit seeds (optional)

1 measure (25ml) of prosecco

Method:

1. Put the ice cubes, water (or juice) and mango into a blender and blitz to a pulp. Add the vodka and lime juice and stir (or shake if you have a cocktail shaker).

2. Pour into a glass (adding more ice if you like) and stir in the passion fruit seeds, if using. Finish with the prosecco over the top.

# Hayley's Cucumber Gin Spritz

This is an exciting twist on the classic G&T, combining two favourite tipples to create a refreshing spritz free of refined sugar.

**Serving suggestion:** in a large wine glass with ice

### All you'll need: (serves 1)

4 Ice cubes

3 cucumber ribbons

1 measure (25ml) of your favourite gin

1 measure (25ml) of prosecco

Soda water

### Method:

1. Put the ice cubes in a glass, add two of the cucumber ribbons, then pour over the gin.

2. Top with the prosecco and finish with soda water and a cucumber ribbon garnish.

# Jaimie's Rum & Ginger Cooler

My friend Jaimie is a beautiful ray of sunshine. She has a gorgeous home in South Africa, but loves to travel and adores the Caribbean. So I created this rum and ginger punch as a little something to bring back those summertime memories for her.

**Serving suggestion:** in a short or tall glass with ice

### All you'll need: (serves 1)

4 ice cubes

1 measure (25ml) of dark rum (or your favourite rum, but dark is best)

Juice of ½ lime

4 mini cubes of peeled fresh ginger

200ml sugar-free ginger ale

### Method:

1. Add the ice to a glass and pour in the rum. Squeeze over the lime wedges, add the ginger cubes and pour in the ginger ale.

2. Stir and enjoy!

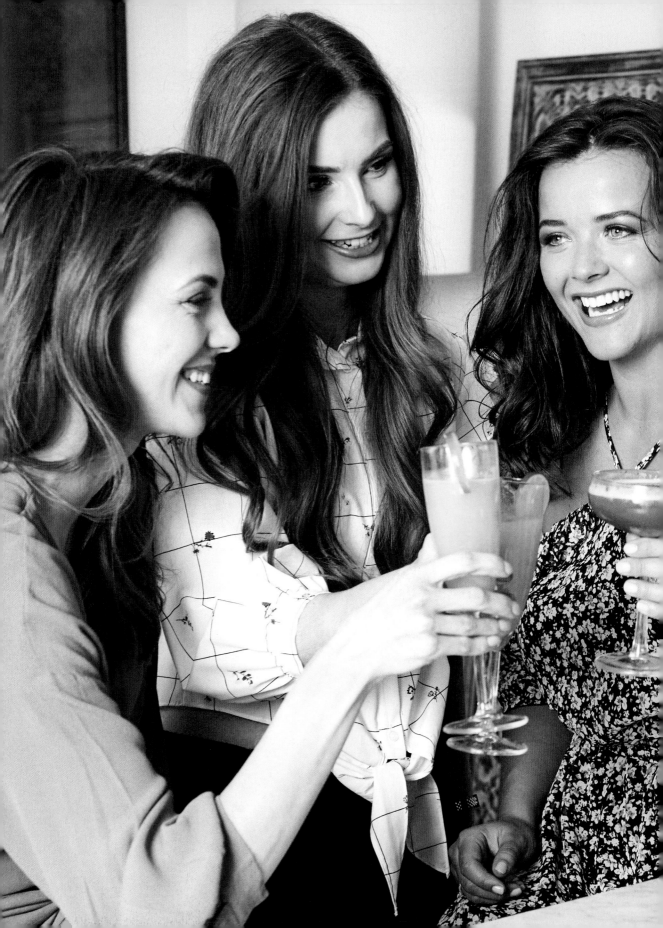

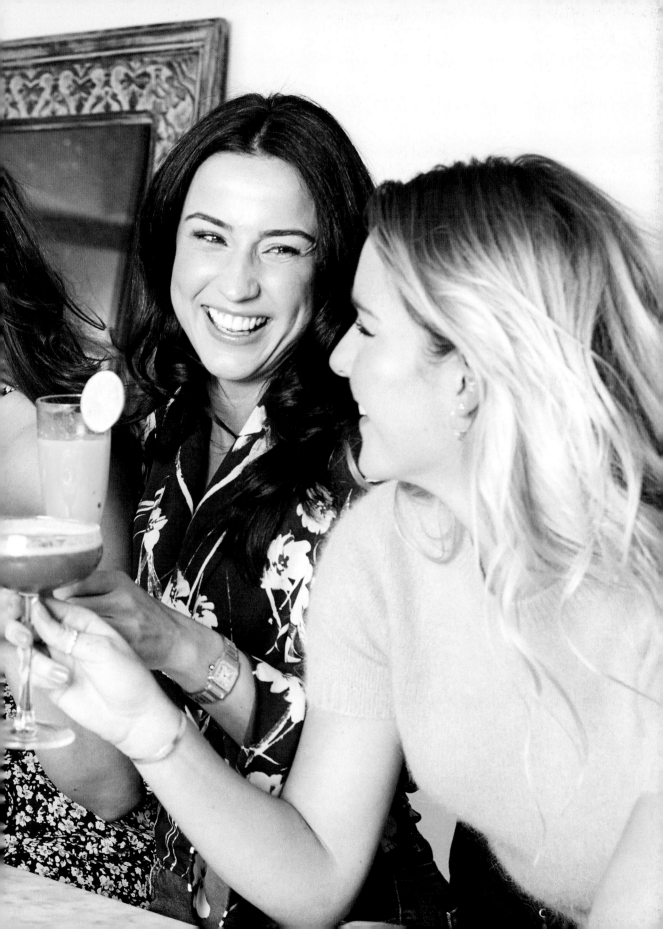

# Letter to You, the Reader...

I wanted to end my story with a heartfelt letter to you. I may or may not know you, but I can honestly put my hand on my heart and tell you that I care about you, your health, your general well-being and your happiness.

I never knew how good healthy truly felt until I allowed myself to embrace it fully, with passion and with strength.

I remember Kate Moss was reported as saying, 'Nothing tastes as good as skinny feels.' Well, I would like to edit that quote by saying, 'Nothing tastes as good as healthy feels.'

This is what I want you to achieve, because I want you to feel as good as I do now. I want you to leave those insecure, unfit, unhealthy, unhappy days behind you and start anew. You deserve it and so does your body.

The only mildly negative thing that has come out of the last year is the fact that my boobs aren't as firm as they used to be, but hey ho! I can live with that, and I can live with the stretch marks too. I have learned that the only thing I can't live without is good health because that is what has brought me true happiness.

On this journey you might find the initial bulk of your excess weight the easiest to lose; I definitely did. The changes I made at first meant that my body lost its excess fat at quite a reasonable pace (12 weeks). Then I had to learn how to maintain my new size 12 frame and to live very comfortably following my new, healthier lifestyle.

At this point, *do not* become complacent; remember, these are choices to be made for life, for your life! The odd hiccup might occur, but you can't expect to reach your dream dress size and then maintain it by going back to old habits.

I have found the last bit of weight the hardest to lose and have realised that it requires me to look more closely into my choices, but my key focus is still my health and making sure that what I do is realistic and sustainable. I just want you to keep a mental note of this because you might experience the same thing.

I also want to remind you that as I write this book, it's only been a year since I began my journey, so it is still ongoing. I love my body as it is, but I will continue to set personal goals to keep me motivated and focused. The most important thing I have achieved is getting my health back; anything else I do now is a bonus and to ensure that I always feel my happiest and most confident.

My message is simple:

Care for your body.

Care for your health.

Respect them.

Love them.

Nourish them.

Your glow and confidence
come from knowing that you are doing all of the above.
They have nothing to do with your shape or
size because those things will take care of themselves.

## LOVE YOUR BODY AND YOU WILL LOVE YOURSELF.

So take this book, use it as the stepping stone to the first chapter in your story and embrace every moment.

With love,

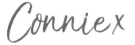

# Acknowledgements

There are so many people I want to thank, not only for giving me the amazing opportunity to share my journey, but also for supporting me and believing in me even before we knew that my journey was going to be such a special thing.

First, I'd like to thank my incredible family, the Simmonds clan – my mum, dad and siblings James, Elliott and Bradley. Thank you for always loving me unconditionally, even when I was miserable, moaning and under the weather. I'm sorry if I made Mykonos a bit crap. Thank you for believing in me, encouraging me and tasting all my recipes. I'm so lucky to have you all in my life.

Bradley, my baby brother, thank you for inspiring me to be the best version of myself and for all of our amazing training sessions. You have helped me beyond belief and in more ways than one; for this I will be eternally grateful.

To my wider family – my grandparents, aunties, uncles, cousins and friends – thank you for being so supportive of me and the incredible year I've had so far. Having such a strong support network has made this an even better experience, so I can't thank you enough.

Tara, Debbie, Hayley and Jaimie – thank you for being a part of my book and joining me for cocktails. That was such a special day and it was amazing to be able to share it with you.

To Ricky, my partner – thank you for making me feel like the most beautiful woman in the world. Every girl deserves a true gentleman like you in her life. You have been there for me regardless of my weight, health, size or mood, and I have never felt anything but loved. Your endless encouragement and support is overwhelming.

A big thank you to my cousin Danielle and the girls at Bare Med Spa (@baremed_spa) for getting me manicure-ready for all the shoots, and thank you to Famida (@famidamua) and Sarah Bridson for hair and make-up on the day. You all made me feel beautiful.

Thank you to my amazing management team, Courtneay Yeates, Issy Lloyd and Natasha at Insanity, for believing in me and my message. I so appreciate all the time and effort you give – it never goes unnoticed – my dream team!

Finally, thank you so much Blink Publishing and Lagom for producing my first-ever book, and to Carly Cook for your unquestioning support throughout the process. I enjoyed every minute. Special thanks also go to the editorial and design team – Ellis, Abi, Mark, Lou and Evee – for all your creativity and for capturing exactly what I had envisioned for *Healthy Forever*. It's such a beautiful book and you are all so talented.

Thanks to all of you, my passion to inspire and motivate women to feel their absolute best from the inside out has been taken to a whole new height, one that I could only have dreamed of without you.